W9-AZT-781

Prevention Effectiveness

Prevention Effectiveness

A Guide to Decision Analysis and Economic Evaluation

Edited by

ANNE C. HADDIX, PHD

STEVEN M. TEUTSCH, MD, MPH

PHAEDRA A. SHAFFER, MPA

DIANE O. DUÑET, MPA

Prevention Effectiveness Activity
Epidemiology Program Office
Centers for Disease Control and Prevention

New York   Oxford
OXFORD UNIVERSITY PRESS
1996

Oxford University Press

Oxford New York
Athens Auckland Bangkok Bombay
Calcutta Cape Town Dar es Salaam Delhi
Florence Hong Kong Istanbul Karachi
Kuala Lumpur Madras Madrid Melbourne
Mexico City Nairobi Paris Singapore
Taipei Tokyo Toronto

and associated companies in
Berlin Ibadan

Copyright © 1996 by Oxford University Press, Inc.

Published by Oxford University Press, Inc.,
198 Madison Avenue, New York, New York 10016

Oxford is a registered trademark of Oxford University Press

All rights reserved. No part of this publication may be reproduced,
stored in a retrieval system, or transmitted, in any form or by any means,
electronic, mechanical, photocopying, recording, or otherwise,
without the prior permission of Oxford University Press.

Library of Congress Cataloging-in-Publication Data
Prevention effectiveness :
a guide to decision analysis and economic evaluation /
edited by Anne C. Haddix . . . [et al.].
p. cm. Includes bibliographical references and index.
ISBN 0-19-510063-8
1. Medicine, Preventive—Evaluation.
2. Medicine, Preventive—Decision making.
3. Medicine, Preventive—Cost effectiveness—Evaluation
4. Medicine, Preventive—Economic aspects.
I. Haddix, Anne C.
RA427.M385 1996 614.4-dc20 95-21249

9 8 7 6 5 4 3 2 1

Printed in the United States of America
on acid-free paper

Foreword

This book, written by the staff at the Centers for Disease Control and Prevention, offers a succinct and pragmatic introduction to the use of cost-effectiveness analysis (CEA) in public health. CEA provides a structure to guide analysts as they evaluate the costs, or resources used, and the effects, or benefits gained, of alternative ways of investing in public health and prevention. With this book as their guide, analysts will be able to apply that structure more fruitfully to inform decision making.

Public health encompasses an astonishing, even bewildering, array of possibilities for improving health—immunizations, control of epidemics, protection of water and food supplies, identification and control of environmental toxins, injury prevention, and the promotion of healthful behavior. As the nation approaches the year 2000, the possibilities for improving health are greater than ever. At the same time, with public spending of all kinds under intense scrutiny, it is more important than ever to ensure that the funds available are serving the nation's highest priority health needs efficiently.

Public health decision makers have always evaluated alternative policies and services, using common sense and whatever methods and data are available and relevant. Epidemiology, the foundational discipline of public health, has provided essential information about the incidence and prevalence of conditions and the likely effects of intervening to improve them, In its 1988 report on the future of public health, the Institute of Medicine urged that evaluation was one of the government's most important public health functions. Government, it stated, must "provide a central mechanism by means of which competing proposals can be assessed equitably."

CEA is a valuable newer tool that serves that function and builds on the basic discipline of epidemiology. Epidemiology is the source of much of the information used to calculate effects. But like public health itself, CEA draws on many disciplines. It adds estimates of costs to those effects. Equally, or more important, CEA provides systematic techniques and approaches that help indicate what information is relevant to an analysis, how to combine it and how to present it. It is a framework for bringing the pieces together to evaluate how well an intervention serves the goals of public health.

CEA calls on a wide range of analytical techniques and data sources, requiring considerable virtuosity on the part of the analyst. This book is written with the understanding that many analysts who need to apply CEA to public health issues do not have time to search out techniques, track down data sources, and make independent evaluations of possible alternatives for the perspective of the analysis, discount rate, and so on. The authors provide practical guidance on these points and others. For example, chapter 3 introduces decision analysis, a valuable organizational as well as analytical tool for CEA. Chapter 5 discusses how to inventory costs, providing worksheets to guide the process. Good sources of data often used in CEA, such as wages, are suggested to save the analyst time and effort.

It is fitting that CDC, the lead federal agency in prevention, has taken the lead here, and not surprising that the book is suffused with an understanding of the practical problems of evaluating public health. One of the most difficult is that, because public-health measures are so wide-ranging, they can have major effects beyond health. Controlling environmental toxins, for example, can affect the price of housing as well as the health of residents. The authors suggest that, when non-health effects are large, cost-benefit analysis may sometimes be a more appropriate technique than cost-effectiveness analysis, because it can combine widely different outcomes in a summary measure of dollar benefits.

One of CEA's principal strengths is that it permits comparisons among interventions. The comparisons can be among closely related alternatives or across a wide range of alternatives, depending on the decision being addressed. Such comparisons are only valid when analyses are conducted in a way to make them so. During the early years of CEA's development, other issues took precedence, but improving the comparability of analyses done by different analysts for different purposes is a logical next step in the development of the method. The CDC has contributed to the enterprise with this volume, which offers many recommendations for grounding analyses in a common set of definitions and assumptions.

In doing so, the book works toward the same goals as the Panel on Cost-Effectiveness in Health and Medicine, a group of thirteen nonfederal experts sponsored by the Public Health Service and co-chaired by me and Milton Weinstein. When it was first convened in 1993, the panel was charged with taking a broad look at CEA with the aim of improving the quality and comparability of studies so that they can contribute to setting priorities among interventions that span the full sweep of health care—public health, prevention, acute care, and rehabilitation. The Panel's work, to be published next year, provides an overview of CEA as well as guidance about its use and future development.

This book shares much in common with the Panel's work. Both, of course, are intended to improve the quality of CEA studies. Both are aimed primarily at analysts, the people who conduct CEA's or supervise their conduct. Users and policy makers are a secondary audience for which the recommendations provide guidance about which analyses are done well and are comparable. Both stress that, in the complex setting in which decisions are made about priorities for public health, and for medicine more generally, CEA is an aid to decision making, not a complete decision-making procedure. Improving the quality and comparability of studies will improve CEA's usefulness as a guide to the many important decisions that must be made in health.

As an analyst and co-chair of the Panel on Cost-Effectiveness in Health and Medicine, I welcome this book and its contribution to the advancement of CEA. Throughout, the book serves the needs of analysts who need to complete good evaluations, useful to the decision at hand, quickly and within a tight budget. They will turn to it often for advice and help.

Louise B. Russell

Preface

As resources have become scarcer and public accountability greater, public health, like clinical medicine, has been forced to re-examine the costs and benefits of its activities as a step in enhancing its ability to allocate resources more effectively. Decision and economic analysis are basic tools in carrying out that mission. These methods have become standard practice in clinical medicine and health services research. This book was written in an effort to apply and adapt that experience to public health situations.

The book was originally written to introduce Centers for Disease Control and Prevention staff to the concepts of decision and economic analysis, to provide guidance on methods to maximize comparability of studies, and to provide access to frequently used reference information. It has been adapted to meet the needs of scientists and managers in state and local health departments and managed care organizations as well as students in schools of public health for an introductory text—a text that shows how these methods can be applied in population-based practice, to facilitate better comparability of studies, and to solidify understanding of the scientific basis for use of these tools in decision making.

HOW TO USE THIS BOOK

Prevention-effectiveness studies have three essential steps: a. framing the study, b. structuring the decision model, and c. analyzing the model and interpreting the results. The steps must be completed in order, and it is especially important that the first two steps are done thoroughly and carefully.

The sequence of chapters in this book follows the sequence of steps outlined above. Each chapter provides an introduction to the methods and options for conducting a prevention-effectiveness study and the basic concepts, underlying principles, and rationales for choosing among alternative approaches. The recommendations presented in each chapter are especially important. Use of the recommendations will increase credibility of the prevention-effectiveness studies and enhance comparability of results across studies.

Prevention effectiveness is the systematic assessment of the impact of piblic health policies, programs, and practices on health outcomes. Chapter 1 provides

an overview of the application of prevention effectiveness to public health problems and introduces the reader to the methodology.

The first step in any prevention effectiveness study, whether a decision
analysis or an economic evaluation, is the framing of the study. This step is
critical to the entire process of prevention-effectiveness reasearch. Chapter 2
identifies thirteen key issues that must be addressed before structuring and
analyzing a problem. Each issue is discussed and recommendations are made
where appropriate. The chapter concludes by providing the reader with a useful
checklist for evaluating a prevention-effectiveness study, protocol, or scope of
work.

Chapter 3 presents the theoretical basis for decision analysis, explains when
and how to do a decision analysis and discuss how to evaluate the results.
Sensitivity analysis is also explained and illustrated. Some benefits of using
decision analysis in public health are also addressed.

Chapter 4 examines the variables embedded in a prevention-effectiveness
decision model. These are the probabilities that link an intervention to a health
outcome. Many of the variables common to prevention-effectiveness models are
identified, including characteristics of the population, screening, preventability,
and risk. The chapter concludes with a catalog of sources for obtaining estimates of variable values.

Chapters 5 and 6 cover costs in economic evaluations. Chapter 5 describes
methods for measuring the cost of prevention interventions for retrospective,
prospective, and modeling studies. A method for estimating intervention costs is
presented including a set of worksheets for cost inventory and analysis. Chapter
6 addresses the issues of adjustments of costs and benefits in a multi-period
model. The methods for discounting, inflating, and annuitizing costs and benefits are presented. Discounting of both monetary and non-monetary costs and
benefits are discussed.

Cost-benefit analysis (CBA) attempts to weigh all the impacts of a prevention
intervention, valued in monetary terms, for the purpose of assessing whether the
benefits exceed the costs. Chapter 7 discusses the theoretical basis for CBA,
describes the method for conducting a CBA within the decision-analytic framework described in the book, and discusses the two most common summary
measures derived from a CBA. Two approaches to estimating the cost of health
outcomes are compared: willingness to pay and cost of illness. Alternative techniques to measure willingness to pay are explored. The chapter concludes with a
discussion of the usefulness and limitations of CBA in evaluating public health
programs.

Cost-effectiveness analysis (CEA) looks at the cost per unit of health outcome
for all intervention options available. CEA is the most frequently used technique
to compare alternative treatment courses or interventions. Chapter 8 addresses
data requirements for conducting cost-effectiveness analyses, provides guidelines for identifying interventions and health outcomes, and discusses interpretation of CEA results. The use of the cost-of-illness approach for estimating
health-outcome costs is presented, including the estimation of medical and

nonmedical costs and productivity losses. The limitations of cost-effectiveness analysis are discussed.

Cost-utility analysis is a special case of cost-effectiveness analysis in which the health outcome is measured in standardized quality adjusted units, such as the "quality adjusted life years" (QALYs). Chapter 9 discusses why and how QALYs are measured, identifies sources of data for measuring quality adjustments, and provides an example of using QALYs in a cost-utility analysis. The usefulness, limitations, and alternatives to the QALY model are also discussed.

A set of appendices follows the main body of the book. These appendices are meant to provide the reader with useful information for undertaking a prevention-effectiveness study. Included in the appendices are a glossary; a catalog of software for decision and economic analysis; two case studies involving decision analysis; a list of sources for cost-of-illness data; a table with 1994 statewide average operating cost-to-charge ratios for urban and rural hospitals; discount and annuity tables; the Consumer Price Index (1960–1994), including the Medical Care and Medical Care Services components; and productivity loss tables. Based on 1990 data and shown by age and gender, these tables are included so that estimation of productivity losses can be standardized in prevention-effectiveness studies. The final two appendices present two important epidemiologic methods for the synthesis of data required in prevention-effectiveness studies. Appendix J covers measures of attribution in prevention-effectiveness research. Derivations and definitions are given for attributable risk and prevented fraction. Appendix K provides an overview of meta-analysis in epidemiologic research. Attention is given to statistical approaches to meta-analysis. Both appendices include a list of references for further study.

As prevention-effectiveness methods are applied with increasing frequency, our understanding of how they can be used most effectively will be refined. We invite readers to comment on this book–content, user friendliness, and orientation–so that we can improve subsequent editions.

Acknowledgments

The editors express their appreciation to William L. Roper, MD, MPH, former Director of CDC, who provided the initial leadership for prevention effectiveness research at CDC.

We also thank the federal and nonfederal experts who reviewed *Prevention Effectiveness: A Guide to Decision Analysis and Economic Evaluation* in its various stages of preparation. A workshop was held in Atlanta, Georgia, April 27–28, 1993, and served as a forum for us to glean ideas from many experts.

We thank the following reviewers: Ward Edwards, PhD; Marthe R. Gold, MD, MPH; Laura Leviton, PhD; Bryan Luce, PhD; Deborah A. McFarland, PhD; Dorothy Rice, PhD; Tanya Roberts, PhD; Louise B. Russell, PhD; Joanna E. Siegel, ScD; George Torrance, PhD; and Milton C. Weinstein, PhD.

We also wish to express our appreciation to the following CDC staff who provided guidance: Suzanne Binder, MD; Edward Brann, MD, MPH; Pennifer Erickson, PhD; Mary E. Guinan, MD, PhD; Susan E. Hillis, PhD, MSN; Thomas A. Hodgson, PhD; Barbara Holloway, MPH; Martha F. Katz, MPA; Ray M. (Bud) Nicola, MD, MSHA; Stephen Ostroff, MD; Dan E. Peterson, MD, MPH; and Stephen B. Thacker, MD, MSc.

While reviewers' comments and suggestions were of tremendous assistance, the authors and editors are responsible for the final content.

Contents

Contributors

SUSAN P. ACKERMAN, PhD, MA
formerly: Acting Chief,
Biometrics & Computer Section
Epidemiology & Statistics Branch
Division of Cancer Prevention and
   Control
National Center for Chronic Disease
   Prevention and Health Promotion, CDC
currently: Vice President
Response Analysis Corporation

HAN CHOI, MD
formerly: EIS Officer
Prevention Effectiveness Activity
Epidemiology Program Office, CDC
currently: Pembroke College
Oxford University

BETH CLEMMER, MPP
Budget Analyst
Financial Management Office, CDC

ERIK DASBACH, PhD
formerly: Health Services Researcher
Division of Diabetes Translation
National Center for Chronic Disease
   Prevention and Health Promotion, CDC
currently: Senior Research Fellow
Merck Research Labs

DIANE O. DUÑET, MPA
Program Analyst
Prevention Effectiveness Activity
Epidemiology Program Office, CDC

PAUL G. FARNHAM, PhD
Visiting Health Economist
Division of HIV/AIDS, CDC
and Associate Professor
Department of Economics
Georgia State University

ROBIN D. GORSKY, PhD[†]
Associate Professor
University of New Hampshire

ANNE C. HADDIX, PhD
Economist
Prevention Effectiveness Activity
Epidemiology Program Office, CDC

ROBERT A. HAHN, PhD
Epidemiologist
Division of Surveillance and Epidemiology
Epidemiology Program Office, CDC

JEFFREY R. HARRIS, MD
Associate Director for Program
   Development
National Center for Chronic Disease
   Prevention and Health Promotion, CDC

DAVID R. HOLTGRAVE, PhD
formerly: Acting Assistant Director for
   Behavioral Science
Office of the Associate Director for HIV,
   CDC
currently: Associate Professor and Director
   of AIDS Policy Studies
Medical College of Wisconsin

†deceased

REBECCA KLEMM, PhD
President
Klemm Analysis Group, Inc.

RICHARD B. ROTHENBERG,
  MD, MPH
formerly: Associate Director for Science
National Center for Chronic Disease and
  Health Promotion, CDC
currently: Director of Preventive Medicine,
Emory University School of Public Health

PHAEDRA A. SHAFFER, MPA
Economic Analyst
Prevention Effectiveness Activity
Epidemiology Program Office, CDC

DIXIE E. SNIDER, MD, MPH
Associate Director for Science
Office of the Director, CDC

DONNA F. STROUP, PhD, MSc
Acting Associate Director for Science
Epidemiology Program Office, CDC

STEVEN M. TEUTSCH, MD, MPH
Chief
Prevention Effectiveness Activity
Epidemiology Program Office, CDC

G. DAVID WILLIAMSON, PhD
Chief
Statistics and Epidemiology Branch
Epidemiology Program Office, CDC

Graphic Artists
PHIL BOURQUE
SANDRA FORD
Epidemiology Program Office, CDC

Editorial Assistance
ELLIOT CHURCHILL, MA
Epidemiology Program Office, CDC

Prevention Effectiveness

1

Introduction

STEVEN M. TEUTSCH
JEFFREY R. HARRIS

Prevention-effectiveness studies involve the systematic assessment of the impact of public health policies, programs, and practices on health outcomes.[1] They scientifically assess the effectiveness, safety, and cost of public health strategies. Their roots lie in the assessment of medical technology and in research on health services and outcomes. Information on prevention effectiveness provides a basis for recommendations regarding public health programs, guidelines for prevention and control, and decision making about resource allocations. Sound decisions require timely, high-quality, comparable, and appropriately directed information. Prevention-effectiveness studies can provide this information.

For many years, particularly in the arena of medical care, it was sufficient to show that the benefits of a technology exceed its hazards before using it. Now in a world of limited resources for public health, officials must use resources as efficiently as possible and must also demonstrate that a technology delivers value for the resources expended.

Prevention-effectiveness studies help meet these goals. They provide a systematic approach to organizing the available information about prevention strategies so that policymakers can have a scientific framework for making decisions. The concept pulls together information from epidemiology and public health surveillance, intervention studies, and economic analyses—using direct evidence when available and indirect evidence when necessary. It addresses basic questions such as

- What is the magnitude of the problem addressed by the prevention strategy? (descriptive epidemiology and public health surveillance)
- Can the intervention work? (efficacy)
- Does the intervention work? (effectiveness)
- What are the benefits and harms of the intervention? (societal perspective)
- What does the intervention cost? (cost analysis)

- How do the benefits compare with the costs? (cost-effectiveness, cost-benefit, and cost-utility analysis)
- What additional benefit could be obtained with additional resources? (marginal and incremental analysis)

CONCEPTUAL MODEL FOR THE DEVELOPMENT OF PREVENTION STRATEGIES

Public health strategies evolve from basic science and applied research through community demonstrations into widespread use (Figure 1.1). The information available at each stage differs, and the methods available for analyzing and synthesizing that information differ as well.

Information on biological risk factors is derived from basic research. Understanding of risk factors focuses attention on initial targets for potential intervention programs. Once major risk factors are identified (e.g., hypercholesterolemia for myocardial infarction or use of seat belts for automobile-crash injuries), applied research, such as randomized controlled trials, is conducted to provide information on the efficacy of an intervention. Research on efficacy shows the degree to which intervention strategies can work under idealized conditions with carefully selected populations and with optimal resources.

After determining which strategies are efficacious, the next step is to deter-

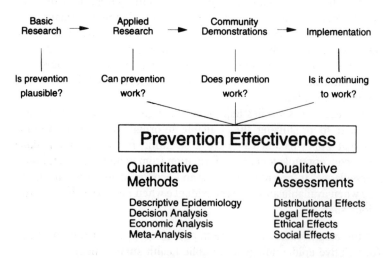

Source: Teutsch, SM. A framework for assessing the effectiveness of disease and injury prevention. *MMWR* 1992: 41 (No. RR-3).

Figure 1.1 Development and implementation of prevention strategies and the role of prevention effectiveness.

mine how well these strategies actually work in community settings. Such community-based demonstrations are used to assess the real-world effectiveness of the prevention strategy. We define effectiveness as the impact that an intervention achieves in the real world under practical resource constraints in an entire unselected population or in specified subgroups of a population. It is axiomatic that effectiveness so defined will almost certainly be lower than efficacy, because of resource constraints, individual compliance, and coverage of an intervention strategy.

Effectiveness research is outcome-oriented. Rather than focusing on the process of disease prevention and control (e.g., measuring how many people receive an intervention), prevention-effectiveness research seeks to link directly the intervention with the health outcome of interest (e.g., mortality, quality of life, or functional status). In this respect, the focus of prevention-effectiveness research differs from that of program evaluation. A prevention-effectiveness study would show, for example, how mortality is decreased by a particular intervention rather than how an intervention was administered.

As prevention strategies are implemented more widely, there is a growing need to maximize the intended impact with the resources available or to obtain a particular impact with as little expenditure of resources as possible. Thus the efficiency of various approaches needs to be examined.

We enter the domain of prevention effectiveness as the results of applied research begin to demonstrate the efficacy of intervention strategies. The process continues throughout the development of the technology into practical public health tools and their application in real settings (see Figure 1.1). Various methods are available for use at each stage of development and implementation.

ATTRIBUTABLE RISK AND PREVENTED FRACTION

In assessing an intervention strategy, one must know what it can realistically accomplish in terms of health outcomes. The first evidence usually comes from research on cause-and-effect relationships associated with health problems, in which the link between a risk factor and an outcome is identified. The relative risk associated with the risk factor provides one measure of the potential impact. However, the overall public health impact is based not only on the relative risk but also on the frequency at which the condition occurs in the population. The impact is measured in terms of attributable risk. The attributable risk is a measure of the amount of disease or injury that could be eliminated if the risk factor never occurred in a given population. It is the maximal limit of disease or injury that could be averted by avoiding a particular risk factor. (In that sense it is analogous to efficacy, i.e., what could be achieved under ideal circumstances.) In contrast, the prevented fraction is a measure of the amount of a health problem that has actually been avoided by a prevention strategy and reflects what can be achieved in a real-world setting. (A more complete discussion of these two concepts can be found in Appendix J.)

PROGRAM EVALUATION RESEARCH AND PREVENTION EFFECTIVENESS

Program evaluation supports prevention-effectiveness research. Program evaluation assesses the processes, impacts, and outcomes of intervention programs, with particular attention paid to the purposes and expectations of stakeholders. Research on evaluation includes a complex array of experimental and quasi-experimental designs. These methods form the basis for determining the effectiveness and efficiency of prevention strategies by providing data on how programs are implemented and consumed.

MODELS FOR PREVENTION EFFECTIVENESS

Models are useful in conducting prevention-effectiveness studies, especially when evidence of effectiveness is indirect or uncertain. In some instances a prevention strategy demonstrably improves a health outcome, and direct evidence of this is available. For example, mammography screening and follow-up for women over 50 years of age have been confirmed to reduce mortality from breast cancer. In many instances, however, such direct effects cannot be measured. When they cannot, indirect evidence of the effectiveness of an intervention must be relied upon. For example, it is known that smoking cessation leads to lowered risk of lung cancer, yet no studies have been conducted that show that a specific smoking-cessation strategy prevents lung cancer. A model would rely on indirect evidence that the smoking-cessation strategy decreases smoking and on the knowledge that cessation decreases the risk of having lung cancer. Such indirect evidence can be used with confidence because each link in the chain of causality can be clearly documented.

Models can be very helpful in making assumptions explicit and in forcing examination of the logic and evidence for each step in the process. The evidence for each step should be assessed using systematic methods and rules of evidence such as meta-analysis (see Appendix K). Although assessments can also include literature reviews or the consensus of experts, such approaches may be subject to bias unless the rules of evidence are followed uniformly.

In addition to structuring effectiveness studies, models are also useful in structuring other types of analyses. Decision analysis (see chapter 3) uses a decision-tree model in comparing alternate strategies. Decision trees include information about the likelihood of each outcome (probabilities) and can incorporate preferences (utilities) or costs or both for different outcomes.

In decision trees and other models, sensitivity analyses permit an assessment of values for which there is uncertainty. Sensitivity analyses can identify critical steps that are likely to make a substantial difference in choosing one strategy over another.

Modeling may also help in identifying the important issues for which data are needed and thereby help to formulate a research agenda; it may also pinpoint issues for which more precise estimates will not affect a decision. Economic analyses are often based on such models. The use of models makes the decision process explicit and can help to clarify the criteria upon which decisions are to be made.

LIMITATIONS

Prevention-effectiveness studies are only tools in the decision-making process. They certainly do not make the decisions themselves. Decision processes should be based on solid technical information such as that obtained from prevention-effectiveness studies, but quantitative information must be combined with an understanding of preferences and values of the stakeholders that are not intrinsically technical in nature. Judgments about those preferences—acceptability, feasibility, and strategic planning—contribute substantially to the decision-making process.

The application of economic analysis in public health is still a relatively new and dynamic area. Although there is general agreement on many of the principles of economic analysis, controversy about their application in public health persists. Thus issues such as choice of discount rates, valuation of life, and discounting of future benefits have not yet been resolved. Because public health economics is an evolving field, researchers are urged to consult economists or decision analysts when they begin to design a study. This collaboration can assure that acceptable methods and current and appropriate data sources are used.

SOCIAL, LEGAL, AND DISTRIBUTIONAL ASPECTS

Although the decision-making aids described in this book can assist in the process of making policy decisions, they are still just aids. Other considerations must also be included in the decision-making process. Many prevention strategies have much broader effects than those directly related to the health outcomes at which they are aimed. This scope of effect is often not included explicitly in the decision-making processes. The social impact of an intervention strategy is well illustrated by the many ramifications associated with human immunodeficiency virus/acquired immunodeficiency syndrome (HIV/AIDS). Intervention strategies implemented for AIDS have raised issues about civil rights among high-risk groups. Sex education and the distribution of condoms in public schools have raised a panoply of concerns reflecting conflicting social values involving students, parents, educators, and public health officials.

It is apparent that prevention strategies must be compatible with the law, but they do raise issues regarding regulations and have an influence on the legal system and precedents. Counseling and testing for HIV/AIDS, for instance, have raised important issues relating to the right to privacy (confidentiality).

Many important advances in public health have required changes in regulations, e.g., limitations on smoking in public places, the work site, or in commercial air travel.

Distributional aspects must also be considered. In the context of limited resources, prevention programs can be focused in different ways. They can be directed intensively toward high-risk populations or, less intensively, toward an entire population. These alternate strategies may have very similar costs and benefits, yet the groups that benefit may differ substantially. Similarly, the group that benefits and the group that is harmed may be different, thus raising issues of equity. For example, fortification of flour with folic acid to prevent neural tube defects is accompanied by the risk of permanent neurological disease because diagnosis of vitamin B12 deficiency may be delayed. The benefits accrue to infants and their families and the hazards to a generally older population. Prevention-effectiveness studies can identify, but cannot resolve, these concerns.

TYPES OF PREVENTION STRATEGIES

Traditional biomedical studies on prevention focus on such clinical strategies to prevent disease and injury as surgical intervention and screening. Prevention-effectiveness studies, however, focus on prevention strategies that encompass the entire domain of public health practice. As a result, many elements of the outcomes and costs are measured differently in prevention-effectiveness studies than they would be measured in clinical prevention studies. In preventing lead poisoning, for example, costs related to a prevention strategy might include the nonmedical costs of removing lead paint from older buildings and replacing plumbing that contains lead in addition to the medical costs of screening and treating persons with elevated blood-lead levels.

Prevention strategies often embody a variety of intervention approaches. In general, however, strategies can be classified as clinical, behavioral, or environmental. Clinical prevention strategies are those conveyed by a health-care provider to a patient, often within a clinical setting (e.g., vaccinations, screening and treatment for diabetic eye disease, and monitoring of treatment for tuberculosis). Behavioral interventions require individual action, such as eating a healthful diet, exercising, stopping smoking, or wearing a bicycle helmet. They may employ a clinical or a population-based implementation strategy. Environmental strategies are those that society can impose and that may require little effort on the part of an individual. Examples of such strategies are laws that limit smoking in public places, dictate the removal of lead from gasoline, prescribe the addition of fluoride to public water supplies, and require the use of seat belts in motor vehicles.

These three approaches should be distinguished from the traditional medical model of prevention based on three stages in disease and injury processes. Primary prevention targets risk factors to prevent occurrence of disease or injury. Secondary prevention targets subclinical disease through early identification and treatment. Tertiary prevention is aimed at established disease or injury to ameliorate progression and maximize function for the person affected.

In keeping with expectations for an introductory text, this book is not intended to be exhaustive, nor does it provide an in-depth theoretical basis for analytic methods. Such information is available elsewhere (see the bibliography at the end of each chapter). A guide to computer software is also included in Appendix B.

Although program evaluation supports prevention-effectiveness research, program-evaluation methods are not specifically addressed in this handbook. Nor do we discuss in depth many social, legal, and distributional issues that are important parts of many policy decisions.

REFERENCES

1. Teutsch SM. A framework for assessing the effectiveness of disease and injury prevention. *MMWR* 1992; 41(No.RR-3):i–iv, 1–12.

BIBLIOGRAPHY

Prevention Effectiveness

Bierman H Jr, Bonini CP, Hausman WH. *Quantitative analysis for business decisions*, 8th ed. Homewood, IL: Irwin, 1991.

Bunker JP, Barnes BA, Mosteller F (eds). *Costs, risks, and benefits of surgery*. New York: Oxford University Press, 1977.

Drummond MF, Stoddart GL, Torrance GW. *Methods for the economic evaluation of health care programmes*. Oxford: Oxford Medical Publications, 1992.

Eddy DM, Hasselblad V, Shachter R. *Meta-analysis by the confidence profile method*. Boston: Academic Press, 1992.

Halperin W, Baker EL, Monson RR. *Public health surveillance*. Boston: Little, Brown & Company, 1992.

Hedges LV, Olkin I. *Statistical methods for meta-analysis*. Boston: Academic Press, 1985.

National Research Council Institute of Medicine. *Toward a national health care survey: a data system for the 21st century*. Washington, D.C.: National Academy Press, 1992.

National Research Council. *Valuing health risks, costs, and benefits for environmental decision making: report of a conference*. Washington, D.C.: National Academy Press, 1990.

Petitti DB. *Meta analysis, decision analysis, and cost-effectiveness analysis: methods for quantitative synthesis in medicine*. New York: Oxford University Press, 1994.

Russell LB. *Is prevention better than cure?* Washington, D.C.: The Brookings Institution, 1986.

Russell LB. *Evaluating preventive care: report on a workshop*. Washington, D.C.: The Brookings Institution, 1987.

Scriven M. *Evaluation thesaurus*, 4th ed. Newbury Park, CA: Sage Publications, 1991.

Sox H, Blatt M, Higgins M, Marton K. *Medical decision making*. Stoneham, MA: Butterworth-Heinemann, 1988.

Stokey E, Zeckhauser R. *A primer for policy analysis.* New York: W. W. Norton, 1978.

Teutsch SM. A framework for assessing the effectiveness of disease and injury prevention. *MMWR* 1992;41 (No. RR-3):i–iv, 1–12.

Teutsch SM, Churchill RE. *Principles and practice of public health surveillance.* New York: Oxford University Press, 1993.

Warner KE, Luce BR. *Cost-benefit and cost-effectiveness analysis in health care: principles, practice, and potential.* Ann Arbor: Health Administration Press, 1982.

Weinstein MC, Fineberg HV. *Clinical decision analysis.* Philadelphia: W. B. Saunders Company, 1980.

Winterfeldt D, Edwards W. *Decision analysis and behavioral research.* Cambridge: Cambridge University Press, 1986.

Economic Analysis

Borus MEJ, Buntz CG, Tash WR. *Evaluating the impact of health programs: primer.* Cambridge: Cambridge University Press, 1982.

Cohen DR, Henderson JB. *Health, prevention and economics.* Oxford: Oxford University Press, 1982.

Drummond MF. Survey of cost-effectiveness and cost-benefit analyses in industrialized countries. *World Health Stat Q* 1985;38:383–401.

Drummond MF, Davies L. Economic analyses along side clinical trials. *Int J Technology Assessment in Health Care* 1991;7(4);561–73.

Drummond MF, Stoddard GL, Torrance GW. *Methods for the economic evaluation of health care programmes.* Oxford: Oxford University Press, 1987.

Eisenberg JM. Clinical economics: a guide to the economic analysis of clinical practices. *JAMA* 1989;262(20):2879–86.

Eisenberg JM et al. Economic analysis of a new drug: potential savings in hospital operating costs from the use of a once-daily regimen of a parenteral cephalosporin. *Rev Infect Dis* 1984;6(4);S909–23.

Feldstein P. *Health care economics,* 3rd ed. New York: John Wiley and Sons, 1988.

Gramlich EM. *A guide to benefit-cost analysis,* 2nd ed. Englewood Cliffs, NJ: Prentice-Hall, 1990.

Harrington W, Krupnick AJ, Spofford WO. *Economics and episodic disease: the benefits of preventing a giardiasis outbreak.* Washington, D.C.: Resources for the Future, 1991.

Hartunian NS. The incidence and economic costs of cancer, motor vehicle injuries, coronary heart disease and stroke: a comparative analysis. *Am J Public Health* 1980;70:1249–60.

Luce BR, Elixhauser A. *Standards for socioeconomic evaluation of health care products and services.* New York: Springer-Verlag, 1990.

Manning WG et al. The taxes of sin: do smokers and drinkers pay their way? *JAMA* 1989;261(11):1604–9.

Mills A. Survey and examples of economic evaluation of health programmes in developing countries. *World Health Stat Q* 1985;39:402–31.

Mohr LB. *Impact analysis for program evaluation.* Pacific Grove, CA.: The Dorsey Press, 1988.

Petitti DB. *Meta analysis, decision analysis, and cost-effectiveness analysis: methods for quantitative synthesis in medicine.* New York: Oxford University Press, 1994.

Rice DP, Hodgson TA, Kopgtein AN. The economic costs of illness: a replication and update. *Health Care Financing Rev* 1985;7:61–80.

Richardson AW, Gafni A. Treatment of capital costs in evaluating health-care programs. *Costs and Management* Nov–Dec 1983;26–30.

Robinson JC. Philosophical origins of the economic valuation of life. *Milbank Q* 1986;64(1):133–55.

Scitovsky A, Rice D. Estimates of the direct and indirect costs of acquired immunodeficiency syndrome in the U.S. 1985, 1986, 1987. *Public Health Rep* 1987;102(1):5–17.

Scitovsky AA. Estimating the direct costs of illness. *Milbank Memorial Fund Q* 1982;60(3):463–91.

Shepard DS, Thompson MS. First principles of cost-effectiveness analysis. *Public Health Rep* 1979;94(6):535–43.

Warner KE, Luce BR. *Cost-benefit and cost-effectiveness in health care.* Ann Arbor: Health Administration Press, 1982.

Weinstein MC, Stason WB. Foundations of cost-effectiveness analysis for health and medical practices. *N Engl J Med* 1977;236(13):716–21.

2

Study Design

PAUL G. FARNHAM
SUSAN P. ACKERMAN
ANNE C. HADDIX

Before beginning a prevention-effectiveness analysis, researchers must address a number of issues. The perspective of the study, the analytic method, and other key issues affect not only the nature of the analysis but the interpretation and usefulness of the results as well. This process is referred to as "framing the question." Its successful completion is one of the most important steps in a study.

This chapter identifies the key points that must be addressed before the analytic process begins, discusses each point, and provides a set of questions that can be used to evaluate a prevention-effectiveness study or protocol. After reading this chapter, the reader should be able to identify answers for each of these key questions as they pertain to a study. Examples are drawn from a variety of prevention-effectiveness studies to show how they might be addressed.

Throughout this and subsequent chapters, recommendations for study design, structure, analysis, and interpretation are embedded in the text. These recommendations are meant to assist in standardizing prevention-effectiveness methodology and increasing the credibility and comparability of studies.

FRAMING THE QUESTION: A LIST OF KEY POINTS

1. Define the *audience* for the evaluation. Identify the users of the results of the analysis, and indicate how the results will be used. Determine the information needs of the target audience in reference to the program or intervention.
2. Operationally define the *problem or question* to be analyzed. This process will influence the types of effects and costs to be included and will help determine which economic evaluation technique is most appropriate for the analysis.

3. Clearly indicate the *prevention strategies* being evaluated, including the baseline comparator (the strategy that best represents current practice) for the evaluation.

4. Specify the *perspective* of the analysis. The perspective taken will determine which costs and benefits are included in the analysis. Limit perspectives to those relevant to the study question.

5. Define the relevant *time frame* and *analytic horizon* for the analysis. Determine the time period (time frame) in which the interventions will be evaluated. Determine how far into the future (analytic horizon) costs and effects that accrue from the intervention will be considered.

6. Determine the *analytic method* or methods. The three methods described in this book are cost-benefit, cost-effectiveness, and cost-utility analysis. The choice of analytic method will depend on the policy question, the outcomes of interest, and the availability of data.

7. Determine whether the analysis is to be a *marginal* or *incremental* analysis. A marginal analysis examines the effect of program scale. An incremental analysis compares the effects of alternative programs.

8. Identify the relevant *costs*. Determine whether the health outcomes will be evaluated using the *cost-of-illness* or the *willingness-to-pay* approach. If the cost-of-illness approach is used, determine whether *productivity losses* will be included. Identify other relevant costs or monetary benefits.

9. Identify the *health outcome* or *outcomes* of interest. Determine whether the outcomes of interest are final health outcomes. The number and nature of outcomes will also help to identify the appropriate analytic method.

10. Specify the *discount rate* or time preference for costs and nonmonetary outcomes that occur in the future.

11. Identify the sources of *uncertainty* and plan *sensitivity analyses*. There may be uncertainty about the effectiveness of a program option in achieving specified health outcomes, or uncertainty about the values of parameters in the model.

12. Determine the *summary measures* that will be reported.

13. If the distribution of the costs and benefits in the population will differ for the prevention-intervention options including the baseline comparator, determine the feasibility of analyzing the *distributional effects* of alternate strategies.

The following sections deal with each of these points in greater detail, including examples and recommendations relevant to various types of prevention programs.

AUDIENCE

The first step in a prevention-effectiveness study is to identify the *audience* for the study. This audience can be defined as the consumers of the study results.

Studies must be framed so that the results will provide information useful for the kinds of decisions that need to be made. Generally, two types of consumers can be identified: policy decision makers and program decision makers. Policy decision makers include elected officials, agency heads, and state and local public health officials. Examples of studies that provide economic data for policy decisions include determining the cost-effectiveness of requiring folic acid fortification of cereal grains to prevent neural tube defects and determining the costs and benefits associated with gasoline additives to reduce carbon monoxide emissions (as mandated by the Clean Air Act).

Program decision makers may use the results of prevention-effectiveness studies to make decisions about different approaches to a prevention program. For instance, an economic analysis for program decision making might determine the most cost-effective smoke-alarm-distribution program to reduce mortality from house fires; it might study whether to implement universal or selected screening for *Chlamydia trachomatis* in public sexually transmitted disease (STD) clinics.

In addition to policymakers and program decision makers, other interested parties may use the results of economic analyses for decision making. These may include managed care organizations, insurance companies, other researchers, patients, health-care workers, the general public, and the press. Identifying the target audience for a study before framing the study question will help to ensure that the analyses conducted provide the information needed by a particular audience in a form useful for that audience.

STUDY QUESTION

Developing a well-constructed and clearly articulated study question is the next step in designing a prevention-effectiveness study. The study question must address the policy or program issues that drive the analysis and must identify the target audience. The study should be framed to reflect the needs of the users of the results of the evaluation. For example, when evaluating the cost-effectiveness of an expanded vaccination program, it may be more useful to ask, "What is the cost-effectiveness of an expanded program versus the current program?" than "What is the cost-effectiveness of the current program versus no program?"

A carefully and clearly stated study question provides the basis for determining other key elements in an economic analysis. Decisions about the perspective of the analysis, the time frame, the analytical method, the costs to be included, and the benefits or outcomes of interest are all determined on the basis of the study question.

INTERVENTION STRATEGIES

Once the study question is clearly defined, the alternate strategies to be analyzed are then selected. These strategies may be apparent from the study question. A sound strategy clearly defines three components: (1) the intervention, (2) the target population for the intervention, and (3) the delivery system. Strategies in the study must be operationally feasible. The availability of data that link the intervention to the health outcome of interest will also determine whether a particular strategy should be included. The lack of evidence of effectiveness may eliminate some strategies from consideration. The analyst must also be careful to select only a limited number of options for the evaluation to prevent the analysis from being too cumbersome, yet must still include all appropriate options so the study provides the information needed for decision making.

In addition to new strategies to be considered, a baseline comparator must also be selected. The baseline comparator may be the existing-program/strategy option or the option of no program if no program exists at the time of the evaluation. The results of the analysis may show that the baseline comparator is the most cost-effective strategy, but this cannot be demonstrated unless it is explicitly included.

Recommendation: The list of alternative strategies in prevention effectiveness studies should include all reasonable options and a baseline comparator (usually either the current program or no program).

PERSPECTIVE

Once the study question has been crafted, the next step is to identify the appropriate perspective or perspectives the analysis will take. Economic analyses typically take the societal perspective—analyzing all benefits of a program (no matter who receives them) and all costs of a program (no matter who pays them). For most public health studies, the societal perspective is appropriate because the goal of the research is to analyze the allocation of societal resources among competing activities. Studies from the perspective of a health-care provider or some other vantage point may be appropriate in such specific instances as those described below.

When an analysis is done from the societal perspective, the costs of a prevention strategy must reflect what members of society give up—now and in the future—to implement the prevention intervention. This is called the *opportunity cost*. Opportunity costs include all program costs regardless of whether they are incurred by an agency, a provider, or a consumer. Thus cost figures may need to be collected for a clinic, a participant, and a public health agency in order to develop a complete measure of program costs. Opportunity costs include more than just the dollar costs associated with providing or receiving health-care services. They also include the resources not available to society because of an illness or injury. If an individual is unable to work, society loses the benefit of that person's contribution in the work force. That loss is described as an opportunity cost. Another opportunity cost would be the value assigned to a person's healthy time that has been forfeited. Because opportunity costs may not appear as a monetary figure in anyone's budget, they may have to be imputed. The opportunity cost of lost work from an illness or injury, also referred to as productivity losses, may be reported separately in the study. In some types of cost utility analyses, the productivity losses associated with the health outcome may have been incorporated into the outcome measure and, therefore, should not be included as a cost. See chapter 9 for a more complete discussion.

In the context of preventing HIV infection, for example, counseling and testing activities at sexually transmitted disease (STD) clinics may be supported by both federal and state funds. When program costs are estimated from the societal perspective, data from both the counseling and testing activities of the program must be collected. Focusing only on the costs incurred by one component may produce a misleading picture of opportunity costs.

Prevention programs that involve outreach into the community may involve volunteers or may have the salaries of some employees subsidized from other sources. *Implicit* or *shadow prices* must be developed for the volunteers' time, and budgetary figures may have to be adjusted to reflect the external subsidies in order to measure these costs accurately from the societal perspective. In addition to time, factors such as transportation, space, materials, telephone, and postage must also be included in total costs. An analysis done from the societal perspective should incorporate all of these costs.

Other Perspectives

The costs and outcomes of prevention programs can also be measured from the perspective of various individuals or groups. Societal costs and benefits, which are relevant for overall resource-allocation decisions, may not be relevant to individuals or organizations that are making a decision about providing or paying for a specific prevention program. Other perspectives include those of (1) *federal, state, and local governments* (the impact on the budgets of specific agencies undertaking a prevention program or on programs such as Medicaid or Medicare, which fund the purchase of health services); (2) *health-care providers* (the costs imposed on various types of hospitals, health maintenance organizations [HMOs], or other providers because of the adoption of particular prevention programs); (3) *business* (the impact of illnesses or prevention activities on health-related employee benefits); and (4) *individuals* (the costs of undertaking a current prevention activity with uncertain future benefits or the costs of illness paid out-of-pocket).

> *Recommendation:* All cost-effectiveness, cost-benefit, and cost-utility analyses (CEAs, CBAs, and CUAs) should take the societal perspective. Additional perspectives may also be studied when relevant to the study question. The perspectives of the analysis should be clearly stated in the introduction of the report of the study.

> *Recommendation:* All measurable opportunity costs, representing all groups that participate in a program or intervention, should be included in the societal perspective.

TIME FRAME AND ANALYTIC HORIZON

The *time frame* of an analysis is the specified period in which the intervention strategies are actually applied. The *analytic horizon* is the period over which the costs and benefits of health outcomes that occur as a result of the intervention are considered. Thus the analytic horizon is often longer than the time frame because the benefits of an intervention may continue after an intervention is completed. Figure 2.1 illustrates the distinction between these two concepts. The figure is based on an example of an intervention delivered over a 1-year period which has a lifetime effect on the individuals who receive the intervention during that year. The lifetime (analytic horizon) effects of chronic heart disease prevented in persons who participate in a cholesterol screening and education program during a 1-year period (time frame) is one such example.

The time pattern of benefits and costs plays an especially important role in economic evaluation of prevention activities. Prevention interventions often occur in the absence of acute health events. Indeed, many years may elapse between the adoption of a type of prevention behavior and the expected development of a health problem that the prevention behavior was designed to prevent. The number of life years gained from a prevention activity may occur far into the future.

It is important to specify a time frame that is long enough to account for several factors: (1) the time frame should be long enough to account for seasonal variations in costs or health outcomes; (2) it should be long enough to have obtained both start-up and ongoing maintenance costs; and (3) it should be long enough to have achieved a steady-state health outcome. As an example, a community bicycle helmet program may initially achieve a sharp increase in the rates at which bicycle helmets are used. As publicity about the program decreases, rates of helmet use may taper off. The time frame for the bicycle helmet

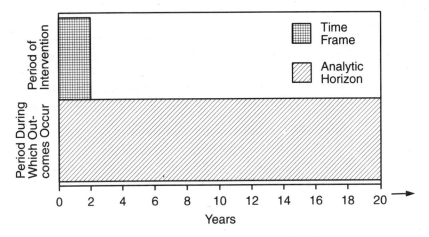

Figure 2.1 The distinction between time frame and analytic horizon.

program should be long enough to temper the effects of the initial publicity about the program and allow an examination of the lasting results of the program. It is often useful to segment the costs and the outcomes of a multiyear intervention to account for the stage of the intervention, e.g., the start-up stage, the early implementation stage, and the maintenance stage.

Although it is important that the time frame of the analysis be of an appropriate length, it should not be overextended. Changes in technology may lead to the obsolescence of a current prevention method within a few years. The choice of time frame should reflect reasonable assumptions about what technology will be used during the time period considered. For example, in evaluating a current screening program such as mammography, if a major new therapy is expected to be available within a few years, a short time frame (perhaps 3–7 years) might be chosen for the analysis. This short time frame should reflect a reasonable assumption about how long the current therapy will still be in use.

Because the time frame for each study must be carefully matched to the intervention being studied, no particular time frame can be generally recommended. However, the time frame of the analysis should always be clearly stated at the beginning of the study.

The *analytic horizon* is the period of time for which costs and benefits related to a particular intervention are measured. Costs may be incurred before an intervention is implemented (e.g., setting up a clinic, training counselors). Costs may also continue after an intervention is implemented (e.g., costs of staff to report statistics). In the case of prevention interventions, benefits are expected to continue after the intervention is completed (e.g., long-term benefits in the form of reduction in high-risk behavior as a result of a specific health education program).

In economic analyses of public health interventions, the ideal analytic horizon is the portion of the lifetime of the persons affected by a prevention intervention, during which time the costs of the intervention are incurred and the benefits are received. An analytic horizon that does not encompass this period may not capture all of the benefits associated with the intervention. If a shorter analytic horizon is selected and some benefits are not captured, the study's comparability with other evaluations of prevention effectiveness is limited. On the other hand, horizons that capture multigenerational benefits, although relevant, may be overly complex and computationally difficult. In some cases, intergeneration effects are crucial. One such case is the evaluation of genetic screening programs for potential parents. For these reasons, the following recommendation is made.

Recommendation: The analytic horizon of an economic analysis should extend over the portion of the lifetime of individuals affected by a prevention intervention, during which time the costs of the intervention are incurred and the benefits are received.

ANALYTIC METHOD

The purpose of an economic analysis in prevention effectiveness is to identify, measure, value, and compare the costs and consequences of alternate prevention strategies. Three methods are commonly used: cost-benefit analysis, cost-effectiveness analysis, and cost-utility analysis. The selection of the appropriate method or methods depends on the target audience for the study, the study question, and the availability of data. In some instances, more than one method may be employed in one study to answer specific policy questions.

Cost-Benefit Analysis

Cost-benefit analysis is a technique that attempts to value the consequences or benefits of an intervention program in monetary terms. The values calculated by this method are measures of the net change in resources expended and gained by a program. Cost-benefit analysis is often used when comparing programs with significant non-health benefits (e.g., enviromental programs which may improve property values). Often, cost-benefit analysis is used to make the decision as to whether to fund a program.

With CBA, program outcomes or benefits are assigned a *monetary value*. Results of a CBA are expressed as net benefits (program benefits minus program costs). The net benefits can then be used in comparing a range of activities with dissimilar measures of health outcome. CBA results indicate whether a specific strategy results in a net gain or net loss. This information can help decision makers select among various programs or among different strategies within a program. Less desirably, results reported in the literature have been expressed as benefit-cost ratios (net benefits divided by net costs). However, because benefit-cost ratios can be distorted, they should not be used. See chapter 7 for a more complete discussion.

Because all costs and benefits are converted into dollar values, CBA raises some controversial questions. What is the exact value of saving one life? Is the life of an older person worth as much as the life of a younger person? Should different values be placed on an outcome that leads to a life with a physical disability and an outcome that leads to a life without disability? If so, does society value persons with disabilities more or less than those who have none? The issues involved with calculating society's willingness to pay to save a life and the use of proxies such as future earnings are discussed in detail in chapter 7.

In summary, the primary disadvantage of cost-benefit analysis for prevention-effectiveness studies is that all benefits are converted to monetary values. Assigning a monetary value to health outcomes—especially the value of a human life—is a difficult and controversial task. The value of averting pain and suffering (classified as an intangible cost) presents a similar problem. Because of the difficulty in measuring and valuing qualitative benefits, prevention-effectiveness practitioners more commonly use cost-effectiveness and cost-utility analysis. However, as our ability to quantify intangibles improves, CBA is becoming a more comprehensive and a more complete measure of changes in societal welfare.

Cost-Effectiveness Analysis

In cost-effectiveness analysis (CEA), no attempt is made to assign a monetary value to health outcomes. Instead of dollars, another measure of outcomes is chosen that is relevant to the question being studied. For example, in comparing programs to promote the use of bicycle helmets, the unit of measure for the CEA might be "head injuries averted." Other units of measures for CEA might include disease prevented or number of lives saved. The unit of measure selected is the outcome most appropriate for the analysis.

Cost-effectiveness analyses are the most commonly performed economic analyses in the health arena. Effectiveness data on outcomes are more generally available and more easily understood than outcome measures for either CBA or CUA. Although CEA uses a unit of measure related to health outcome, CEA still considers the costs of a program and the costs saved by the program (the net cost). Operationally, it is defined as the net cost divided by the net effectiveness (see chapter 5 for more details).

CEA combines the net cost of implementing an intervention with the effectiveness of the intervention. Results are expressed in various ways depending on the health outcome selected, e.g., CEA results might be stated as "cost per life saved" or "cost per injury averted."

Cost-effectiveness analysis is most useful when the goal is to identify the most cost-effective prevention strategy from a set of alternate interventions that produce a common effect. The disadvantage of cost-effectiveness analysis is that because there is no single type of outcome, the comparability of cost-effectiveness studies for different health conditions is limited. Also, because the value to society of a life and the quality of life beyond the value assigned to a person's economic contribution is not included in a CEA, judgments about the value and quality of lives must be made implicitly by the user of the study results.

Cost-Utility Analysis

Cost-utility analysis (CUA) is a variant of cost-effectiveness analysis. CUA allows prevention strategies for more than one disease or health problem to be compared. In cost-utility analysis, as in cost-effectiveness analysis, a common measure is used to compare alternate strategies. In CUA, net benefits are expressed as number of life years saved, with a quality-of-life adjustment. Thus, the common measure for CUA is quality-adjusted life years.

The measure of quality-adjusted life years has an intuitive appeal to decision makers. Rather than relying on implicit judgments about the value and quality of life, CUA makes these values explicit in the calculation. However, quality-adjusted life years are subjective determinations, are difficult to measure, and are not universally accepted.

CBA, CEA, and CUA are methods appropriate in different circumstances.

The availability of data, the way a study question is framed, and the information needs of the audience all influence the selection of the type of analytic method. In addition, the selection of an analytic method or methods is also linked to the selection of outcome measures, discussed below.

CBA, CEA, and CUA utilize data and methods described in subsequent chapters. Cost-benefit analysis is described in more detail in chapter 7, cost-effectiveness analysis in chapter 8, and cost-utility analysis in chapter 9. Specific recommendations regarding the use of these methods are found in these chapters.

MARGINAL AND INCREMENTAL ANALYSIS

Marginal analysis examines the effect on health outcomes of making an additional investment in an intervention. For example, determining the cost-effectiveness of spending an additional $2 million in a cereal grain fortification program to double the folic acid level to prevent neural tube defects requires a marginal analysis, because the policy question addresses the effect of adding additional resources to one intervention.

In contrast, incremental analysis examines the relationship between making an investment in a different intervention and the health outcomes expected to be produced by that strategy. Determining whether fortification of cereal grains is a more cost-effective strategy to prevent neural tube defects than a vitamin supplementation program requires an incremental analysis.

Marginal and incremental analyses are fundamental to prevention-effectiveness studies. They are the basic foundation of the comparative measures used to decide among strategies.

Average costs are a poor substitute for marginal and incremental costs. Average costs provide information about only a particular strategy. Marginal and incremental costs allow for comparison among strategies and ranking them by their marginal returns.

Recommendation: Marginal or incremental analysis should always be performed in a prevention-effectiveness study. The results of marginal and incremental analyses should be reported. Discussion should include the interpretation and the implications of the marginal or incremental results.

COSTS

It is useful to identify all relevant costs in the evaluation before constructing the model. The availability of data on cost may affect decisions about the perspective of the analysis and the analytic method. Sources of data on cost should also be identified. Chapters 5 and 6 contain a complete treatment of intervention cost collection and analysis. The willingness-to-pay approach to estimating the monetary value of health outcomes and other benefits is included in chapter 7.

The cost-of-illness approach to measuring the medical costs and productivity losses averted is presented in chapter 8. A list of data sources for costs is provided in Appendix E.

OUTCOMES

In prevention-effectiveness studies, outcomes are the results of implementing a prevention strategy. Outcomes are usually considered in terms of health conditions, e.g., quality-adjusted life years or cases prevented. The first is an outcome measure that would be used in a cost-utility analysis. The second outcome measure would be more frequently used in a cost-effectiveness analysis. The value of either, expressed in monetary terms, as well as the value of other outcomes not related to health would be used in a cost-benefit analysis.

Not only is the selection of outcome measure guided by the analytic method used, it is also guided by the policy question to be answered and by the kind of data that can reasonably be collected. Lack of data to conduct a particular type of analysis may make it necessary to select another analytic method and another, perhaps less preferable, outcome measure. For example, in a recent study of the cost-effectiveness of programs to promote the use of bicycle helmets among children, it was determined that the use of quality-adjusted life years saved would best answer the policy question, because this would allow both fatal and nonfatal head injuries to be included in one measure. However, data did not exist on the severity of the head injuries; only data regarding the number of head injuries were available. Thus it was not possible to use a quality-adjusted measure. Because of this, two outcome measures were selected: head injuries prevented and fatalities prevented. Cost-effectiveness ratios were calculated for each.

For many public health prevention strategies implemented outside the clinical arena, benefits other than health outcomes may also be of interest. For example, in a recent study of the impact on health of the installation of municipal water and sewer systems in *colonias* on the U.S.–Mexico border, one of the primary benefits was an increase in property values. Without taking this benefit into account as one of the outcomes, the study would fail to convey the full measure of benefits of the program. Therefore, it was decided that a cost-benefit analysis would best capture both economic and health benefits in a single summary measure.

A more complete discussion of selection and measurement of outcomes is included in the chapters on analytic methods.

DISCOUNT RATE

Time affects the monetary valuation of program outcomes and costs because individuals generally weigh benefits and costs in the near future more heavily than those in the distant future. A dollar that an individual receives this year is worth more than a dollar that will be received 10 years from now. This is because this year's dollar can be invested so in 10 years' time it will be worth more than a dollar. This argument also applies to the valuation of capital and investments. It may also be worth more now because the individual prefers to make purchases today than postpone consumption until the future. This concept is referred to as *time preference.* As a rule, the societal preference is for health benefits received today versus health benefits received in the future. See chapter 6 for a more complete discussion.

The discount rate used in prevention-effectiveness studies is not related to inflation. Even in a world of zero inflation, the value of a dollar received today would be greater than the value of a dollar received in the future (see chapter 7). Using a discount rate in an economic analysis provides a method of adjusting the value of receiving benefits today versus receiving benefits in the future or of incurring costs in the present versus incurring costs in the future.

Since most public health projects involve benefits and costs that continue into the future, it is necessary to calculate the present value of these benefits and costs to make them comparable in terms of the time dimension. This calculation of present value involves the choice of a discount rate. The choice of a discount rate is a controversial issue that can have a significant impact on the results of the analysis. This issue is explored in greater depth, and recommendations about specific discount rates and discounting of health outcomes are given in chapter 6.

UNCERTAINTY

Often in prevention-effectiveness studies, precise estimates are not available for certain variables. This may reflect limitations of previous studies or the fact that studies in different population settings have yielded a range of estimates. The initial assumptions made about a study definitely influence its results. It is important to list in the study all of the assumptions upon which the values of variables are based.

Recommendation: All assumptions should be explicitly stated in the study, including assumptions about the structure of the decision model and the probabilities, outcome measures, and the costs in the decision model.

Sensitivity-analysis techniques and interpretation are covered in more detail in chapter 3.

SUMMARY MEASURES

A number of summary ratios can be reported in a prevention-effectiveness study. As noted earlier, it is important to identify the outcome measures that most accurately address the study questions before beginning an analysis. Once the outcome measures have been identified, the decision analysis can then be structured with the desired output in mind. However, regardless of the analytic method used, a marginal or incremental analysis should be performed, as described above. The marginal or incremental measure should then be used as a primary summary measure for the study.

Examples of summary measures include the incremental net present value of benefits (CBA), the incremental cost-effectiveness ratio (CEA), and the incremental cost-utility ratio (CUA). Average summary measures may also be reported but should not be used to compare prevention strategies. Summary measures and their calculations are discussed in detail in chapters 7, 8, and 9.

DISTRIBUTIONAL EFFECTS

As discussed in the introduction, the way a prevention intervention is implemented may affect the distribution of costs and benefits. "Who pays the most?" and "Who receives the greatest benefit?" are questions with legal, ethical, political, and practical implications. Policymakers should consider distributional effects when making decisions about prevention programs.

In economic analyses, identification of the potential shifts in distribution of costs is useful in ensuring the collection of appropriate data and in the classifying of costs and benefits for the study. Examination of subpopulations or the selection of an additional perspective for the analysis may be based on potential distributional effects.

Recommendation: When possible, the distributional impacts of a study should be examined. This investigation may be limited to discussion of the possible implications of the results of the study but may include more detailed analysis of direct impacts using a disaggregated study population.

COMPARABILITY OF THE STUDY RESULTS

It is extremely important for persons who conduct prevention-effectiveness studies to make clear all of the assumptions about the factors discussed in this chapter. Study results should be reported with all assumptions explicitly identified including audience perspective, outcome and cost measures, use of discounting, and discount rate.

Unfortunately, this policy has not always been followed in the studies currently reported in the literature. A review of 77 cost-effectiveness and cost-benefit studies in the medical literature indicated that only 18% of the studies explicitly stated what perspective the analysis used, with the rest leaving the determination of the perspective to the readers.[1] The lack of clear definition of assumptions seriously compromises the scientific integrity of a study and makes the results virtually useless for comparison purposes.

Economic analyses of prevention programs should also indicate the robustness of their results through the use of sensitivity analysis or other techniques.

Because studies incorporate a wide variety of assumptions and data of inconsistent quality, users of the study need to know which assumptions and data are the most important to the overall results. Users can then incorporate their own estimates of these factors if they are not satisfied with the decisions made or assumptions used in the analysis.

CONCLUSION

The key points discussed above are essential for conducting and evaluating prevention-effectiveness studies. Each of the key points may have a substantial impact on the results of an analysis. Not only should they be addressed in conducting a study, they should also be clearly reported. A checklist of key points follows.

CHECKLIST FOR EVALUATING THE PROTOCOL OR SCOPE OF WORK FOR A PREVENTION-EFFECTIVENESS STUDY

1. Was the audience for the study clearly identified?
2. Was the study question clearly defined? Did the question follow a clear description of the public health problem?
3. Were the alternate prevention strategies clearly identified and described? Was a baseline comparator included as a strategy?
4. Was the perspective of the analysis stated? Will the analysis take a societal perspective? Will a more limited perspective also be taken?
5. Were the time frame and the analytic horizon defined? What is the time period over which the alternative strategies will be evaluated? Over what period of time will the costs and benefits of health outcomes that occur within the intervention time frame be measured?
6. Were the analytic method or methods specified? Will the study use a cost-benefit, cost-effectiveness, or cost-utility analysis? Will a marginal or incremental analysis be conducted?
7. Were the costs clearly identified? Were the costs of the alternate strategies included? Will the study take the cost-of-illness or willingness-to-pay approach to measuring the value of health outcomes or adverse health effects? If the cost-of-illness approach is chosen, will productivity losses be included? Were other relevant costs included (e.g., cost to government, business)?
8. Was the health outcome clearly identified? Are there multiple outcomes? Are the outcomes final outcomes?
9. Was the discount rate specified? Will sensitivity analysis be conducted on the discount rate?
10. Were the sources of uncertainty in the model identified? Will appropriate sensitivity and threshold analysis be conducted?
11. Were the summary measures identified?

12. Will the distributional effects of the alternate strategies be examined?

REFERENCES

1. Udvarhelyi IS, Colditz GA, Rai A, Epstein, AM. Cost-effectiveness and cost-benefit analyses in the medical literature. *Ann Intern Med* 1992; 116: 238–44.

BIBLIOGRAPHY

Barry PZ, DeFriese GF. Cost-benefit and cost-effectiveness analysis for health promotion programs. *Am J Health Promotion* 1990; 4:448–52.

Drummond MF, Stoddart GL, Torrance, GW. *Methods for the economic evaluation of health care programmes.* Oxford: Oxford University Press, 1987.

Lave JR, Lave LB. Cost-benefit concepts in health: examination of some prevention efforts. *Prevent Med* 1978; 7:414–23.

Murphy RJ, Gasparotto G, Opatz, JP. Methodological challenges to program evaluation. *Am J Health Promotion* 1987; 1:33–40.

O'Donnell MP, Ainsworth TH. *Health promotion in the workplace.* New York: John Wiley and Sons, 1984.

Russell LB. *Is prevention better than cure?* Washington, D. C.: The Brookings Institution, 1986.

Russell LB. *Evaluating preventive care.* Washington, D. C.: The Brookings Institution, 1987.

Udvarhelyi IS, Colditz GA, Rai A, Epstein, AM. Cost-effectiveness and cost-benefit analyses in the medical literature. *Ann Intern Med* 1992; 116: 238–44.

Warner KE. The economic evaluation of preventive health care. *Soc Sci Med* 1979; 13C: 227–37.

Warner KE, Luce, BR. *Cost-benefit and cost-effectiveness analysis in health care.* Ann Arbor: Health Administration Press, 1982.

3
Decision Analysis

DIXIE E. SNIDER
DAVID R. HOLTGRAVE
DIANE O. DUÑET

As discussed in chapter 2, the framing of a prevention-effectiveness study provides the foundation for the entire process of conducting prevention-effectiveness research. Once the study has been appropriately framed, a problem can begin to be structured. Decision analysis is one technique that is frequently used for this process. Decision analysis can function as either a "stand-alone" method for decision making or as a framework for conducting CBAs, CEAs, and CUAs. This chapter provides an overview of the process of decision analysis.

This chapter covers the following topics:

- The theoretical basis for decision analysis
- When to do a decision analysis
- How to do the basic steps of decision analysis
- How to evaluate the results and harness uncertainty
- Common criticisms of decision analysis
- Possible benefits of using decision analysis in public health

Case studies presented in Appendix C and Appendix D illustrate the process of structuring a problem and constructing a decision-tree model. The reader is encouraged to work through the case studies to clarify and expand the concepts presented elsewhere in the book.

DECISION ANALYSIS DEFINED

Decision analysis is an explicit, quantitative, and systematic approach to decision making under conditions of uncertainty. Decision analysis complements, but does not replace, professional judgment or expertise. It is a philosophy and methodology for making decisions. Decision analysis provides a framework for decision making based on what is known, what can be done, and what is preferred.

Many decisions have an important impact on public health and medical practice. Deciding to support a program with funding, setting priorities on research areas, or making recommendations on screening and treatment are important decisions with potentially far-reaching impact. Decision making is often complex. Many times, decision makers must operate without complete information and research data; in the context of competing priorities; and under political, policy, and time constraints.

THEORETICAL BASIS FOR DECISION ANALYSIS: EXPECTED UTILITY

The foundations of decision analysis were set in place during the 1700s with Bernoulli's work on expected utility theory.[1] Since that time, the field has been "rediscovered" several times. The publication of the second edition of von Neumann and Morgenstern's *Theory of Games and Economic Behavior* in 1947,[2] usually considered a contribution to economic theory, is often said to have established decision analysis as a modern field of study. During the late 1950s and early 1960s, the fundamental concepts of decision analysis were developed. Robert Schlaifer is credited with publishing the first textbook on the subject, *Probability and Statistics for Business Decisions* in 1959.[3] The term *decision analysis*, however, was not used until 1966, when R. A. Howard published an article called "Decision analysis: applied decision theory."[4] By 1959, efforts had begun to apply the theoretical concepts of decision analysis to real-world problems, including health problems[5]; however, medical applications of the new science did not appear in the literature for nearly a decade.[6] Since the early 1970s the application of decision analysis to medical problems has burgeoned. The journal *Medical Decision Making* was established in 1981 to provide a forum for both theoretical and practical developments in the field. Decision analysis has been applied to the study of public health since the 1980s. Today it is an accepted and widely used method for examining public health policy.

Decision analysis uses mathematical tools to help decision makers choose the option that maximizes utility. *Utility* is defined as the value of a preferred outcome when considered from a particular perspective. Thus decision analysis can be viewed as a technique for helping decision makers identify the option that has the greatest expected utility to an individual, to society, or to a particular community.

The decision-analytic framework used to calculate expected utility can also be used to calculate cost-effectiveness in CEAs and net present value in CBAs. Such models do not explicitly include utility as the value of an outcome but are used to calculate the expected cost and benefit and enumerate expected outcomes (CEA) of the options in the decision tree. Models for CBA and CEA are based on different theoretical foundations, but the techniques for working with such models do not differ.[7]

The study of making decisions can be divided into three areas: descriptive models, normative models, and prescriptive techniques. *Descriptive models* are used to explain and predict how decisions are made. For example, studies of group behavior and descriptive decision-making models can be used to predict the choices a group will make in a particular situation.

Normative models provide rules by which decisions *should* be made. Normative models use logic and other rational bases for choosing among options. Some organizations adopt normative decision models as policies for making routine decisions. For example, when confronted with various budget options, the choice of the one that maximizes the number of lives saved may become a decision rule formalized as an organizational policy.

In real life, most decisions are not made using the particular logic and rationality of decision analysis. When the way people *actually* make decisions differs from the way people *should* make decisions, *prescriptive techniques* of decision analysis may be useful. Prescriptive techniques help move people toward normative rules for decision making and help organize and clarify the decision-making process.

The basis for the normative technique of decision analysis discussed below is based on both expected-utility theory and the theory of welfare economics. Expected-utility theory assumes that, given different options, the one with the outcome that has the highest *expected utility* should be chosen. Expected utility is calculated from estimates of the probability of possible outcomes and the strength of preference for a specific outcome. Thus, decision analysis provides a systematic way of identifying choices, quantifying expectations or probabilities, assigning values to possible outcomes, and comparing options. The preferred option is selected based on a predetermined decision rule.

WHEN TO DO A DECISION ANALYSIS

Use Decision Analysis for Other than "Everyday" Decisions

Decision analysis is not needed for making most decisions, because the decision topic is trivial, because the most desirable option is obvious, or because the available choices lead to outcomes with equal or nearly equal value. For example, it may not make much difference whether one chooses to have an orange or an apple with lunch. A person may not care a great deal about whether to borrow money from a bank or some other type of lending institution, but if one bank lends money at 9% interest and another at 12%, the borrower will have no trouble recognizing that it is preferable to borrow from the bank that charges lower interest.

Even in making complex decisions, people seldom use the tools of decision analysis. Decision making may require the collection and integration of large amounts of complex, imperfect information. Rather, to deal with complex decisions, people often rely on psychological shortcuts in thinking called *heuristics*. Heuristics can be useful by helping to simplify complex decisions. However, some heuristics can lead to suboptimal choices.[8]

To simplify the task of making difficult decisions, decision analysis can be used to help structure the decision-making process. Decision analysis provides a way to approach a decision in a logical manner and to incorporate the short- and long-term consequences of the various options.

Use Decision Analysis When the Choice Is Not Clear

Even in a complex situation, sometimes one choice is clearly preferable to all others, and it is easy to decide what to do. In such cases, decision analysis may help to document the basis for the choice made, but an analysis really does not help the decision-making process. Decision analysis may take considerable time and effort. If there is already an answer with which everyone feels comfortable, a decision analysis is not necessary.

Use Decision Analysis When Real Choices Exist

Decision analysis should be done only when there are real options to consider. Sometimes there may be only one real choice available. "Options" that are illegal, unethical, too expensive, or unavailable are not real choices. Thus it is a waste of effort to do a decision analysis to choose among these nonchoices.

Use Decision Analysis in Close-Call Situations and When Consequences Are Important and Sweeping

Decision analysis is most useful in "close-call" situations, when real choices exist and when it is not clear which choice to make. When the consequences of a decision are important and sweeping, decision analysis can be an important step in the decision-making process. Vaccination programs, long-term treatment programs, and programs requiring a substantial investment in infrastructure require careful analysis even when one option intuitively seems clearly preferable to all others.

BASIC STEPS IN DECISION ANALYSIS

There are several approaches to decision analysis including decision-tree models, influence diagrams, and the analytic hierarchy approach. Decision analysis using decision trees is the method most widely accepted and easily adaptable to prevention-effectiveness research. The decision-tree method of decision analysis is recommended as one method for use in prevention-effectiveness studies. For simplicity, throughout this book *decision analysis* will refer to decision analysis using a decision-tree model.

The six basic steps in decision analysis are

- Structuring the problem
- Developing a decision tree

- Estimating probabilities
- Valuing consequences
- Averaging-out-and-folding-back
- Interpreting results in light of inherent uncertainty

Structuring the Problem

Structuring a problem is the first step in decision analysis. Depending on how the problem is structured, the decision analysis can give relevant, meaningful answers or it can mislead the decision maker. With the computer software currently available, it is tempting to rush ahead with a computer-based decision-analysis program. However, organizing and structuring a problem is the basis for the entire decision analysis, and it should be done carefully. Otherwise the decision analysis may produce a sophisticated solution to the wrong problem or to an inadequately structured problem.

Problem structuring leads to a clear statement of the major issues involved in a decision. It can also be useful in itself. In the process of problem structuring, objectives are clearly defined; alternatives are identified and reformulated; and areas of agreement and disagreement among decision makers become clearer. Sometimes problem structuring is all that is needed for a decision maker to be able to make a choice.

To structure a problem, the following questions need to be answered:

- What are the major issues involved in the decision?
- What is the perspective of this analysis?
- What are the real alternatives?

Stating the Major Issues

A problem should be stated clearly in a way that targets the ultimate question to be answered. It is important to consider the underlying questions and issues at the core of a problem and to be sure that the analysis approaches the problem at the appropriate level. For example, is the question whether to implement a condom-distribution program versus a media-based education program, or is the question whether to implement an education program that is school- or mass-media-based?

Defining the Perspective

Depending on the viewpoint taken in the initial stages of the problem structuring, the resulting questions may lead to different analytic answers. If a decision maker takes the perspective of an individual at risk for complications following pregnancy, the problem structure might look different from the way it would be viewed by society at large. Public health decisions may involve the viewpoints of communities, nations, individuals, interest groups, agencies, programs, and others.

In structuring a problem, a viewpoint may sometimes be prescribed by an outside source. For instance, if the U. S. Congress requests information about program efficiencies and justification of proposed programs, a national perspective may have to be included in the decision analysis. In another area, certain aspects of problem structuring may be inherent in the mission of an organization. For example, a chronic disease program may be choosing among chronic-disease-prevention programs rather than choosing between chronic- and infectious-disease-prevention programs. In these cases, the problem structures would begin with certain boundaries.

Identifying Options
Next, options should be identified. Only those that have the possibility of being implemented should be included in the problem structure. In this process, any options that are not really being considered should not be included. Conversely, all viable options should be included.

Considering the Analytic Horizon
An essential step in structuring a problem is deciding how far into the future to consider the outcomes of a decision. In the case of childhood vaccinations, for example, the analytic horizon from childhood to death in old age would add to the complexity of the decision analysis. Sometimes an analytic horizon can be shortened to simplify the modeling involved; however, one must be careful not to exclude substantial costs and benefits that may occur in the future. In any case, it is important to decide on a logical stopping place when structuring a decision problem and deciding on an analytic horizon.

Developing a Decision Tree

A decision tree is a graphic representation of how all the possible choices relate (stochastically) to the possible outcomes. The term *decision tree* is used because options are arranged to resemble a tree in appearance. A decision tree is typically sketched out by hand in several versions. Although a decision maker or decision analyst may attempt to devise a decision model independently, in optimal circumstances a decision tree is derived through collaboration by a decision team, who come to some agreement on the decision options and the structure of the problem as represented by the tree.

A *decision option* is defined as a possible choice among all options. Each possible choice that is included in the decision analysis is called a decision option. As a starting place for constructing the decision tree model, each decision option should be listed.

The first point of choice in the decision tree is represented by a *decision node* (usually drawn as a square). Each decision option is represented by a line attached to the box (Figure 3.1). At this decision node, the only alternatives are "vaccinate" and "do not vaccinate." Only one of these options is to be chosen.

Regardless of which decision option is chosen, an individual's final outcome is determined by a series of chance events. Even if a person is vaccinated, there is a chance (probability) that the person may still contract disease. In the case of "do not vaccinate," there is a certain probability that a person may not get the

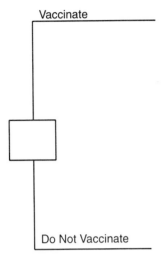

Vaccinate

Do Not Vaccinate

Figure 3.1 Two alternatives in a decision tree.

disease even though that person did not receive the vaccine. (The assignment of probabilities is discussed in the next section.) In the creation of a decision tree, an event whose outcomes are not under the control of the decision maker is denoted by a chance node (symbolized by a circle). Figure 3.2 shows two chance nodes. Each outcome of a chance event is denoted by a line attached to the circle. Each line is labeled with the name of the outcome. Then, for each decision alternative, a numerical probability must be assigned that represents the chance that an individual will have a particular outcome.

The decision tree is usually written from left to right, starting with the initial decision node on the extreme left and moving to the final outcomes on the extreme right. The sequence of chance nodes from left to right in the decision tree usually follows the temporal sequence of events. A *terminal node*, represented by a box, indicates the end point of each sequence of events. Expanding the vaccination example from above, Figure 3.3 shows how each option progresses through time. Although the decision tree in Figure 3.3 shows just two or three outcomes at each chance node, there is no limit on the number of outcomes at a chance node. One rule is important: the events at a chance node must be *mutually exclusive and exhaustive.* All possible events must be listed, and there must be no overlap in the definition of these events.

Estimating Probability

The next step in creating a decision tree is assigning a probability to each event that is controlled by chance. Probability estimates can be obtained from literature searches, results of scientific studies, estimates made by panels of experts, or the use of ranges of probabilities. (For a further discussion of probability ranges, see "Harnessing Uncertainty" below.)

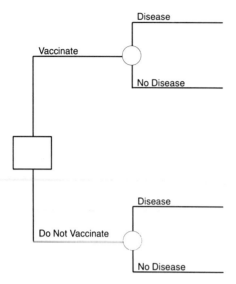

Figure 3.2 Chance nodes in a decision tree.

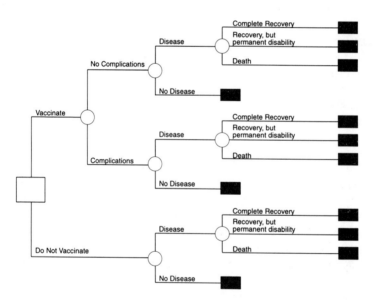

Figure 3.3 Terminal nodes in a decision tree.

At each chance node, the numerical value of an estimated probability is noted on the decision tree. Because the events at each chance node must be mutually exclusive and exhaustive, *the sum of the probabilities at each chance node must equal 1*. Using the vaccination example, Figure 3.4 shows the decision tree with hypothetical probability values inserted.

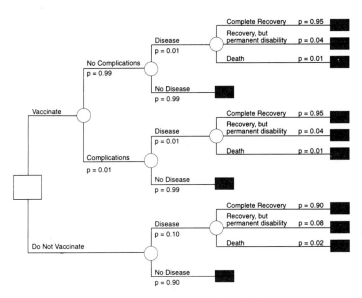

Figure 3.4 Probabilities at chance nodes in a decision tree.

Valuing Consequences

The next step in the decision analysis is to assign a value to each outcome on the decision tree. For some analyses, appropriate units of measure may occur naturally. For example, units of cost or effectiveness may be used as a quantitative measure of the value of an outcome in a decision tree. If a decision is to be made on the basis of costs or such other known values as effectiveness, then these values may simply be inserted in the decision model to correspond with each possible outcome.

For other analyses, assigning values to decision-tree outcomes is not as straightforward because no natural units of measure are available. In these cases, a scale of utility values must be devised. Utility is a quantitative measure of the strength of preference for an outcome. All outcomes are not of equal value. For instance, an outcome of health would be preferred to an outcome of death. Estimating utilities allows the decision maker to factor in preferences for certain outcomes and to distinguish among complex outcomes (e.g., immediate death, death after long suffering, death after no suffering, no death). There are two aspects of estimating utilities: choosing a method for estimation and choosing a common scale.

When quantitative outcomes are used, e.g., the cost of a medical outcome or a case of disease prevented, the *expected values* for the decision alternatives are calculated. When the outcomes are qualitative measures, e.g., utilities, the *expected utilities* for the decision alternatives are calculated. The same calculation is performed for both expressions.

Valuing Outcomes
A simple method for valuing outcomes is called *rank and scale*. In this method,
outcomes are ranked in order of best to worst and then are assigned numerical
values. For example, at one chance node, three outcomes might be possible and
might be ranked as follows:

Complete recovery   8
Recovery with disability   5
Immediate death   0

In this example, the value of "5" is a subjective judgment. There are many
other, more sophisticated methods for valuing outcomes. Chapter 9 describes
estimating utilities in terms of quality-adjusted life years.

Choosing a Common Scale
Usually the value of an outcome is affected by a variety of attributes, such as
personal preferences and perceived usefulness of an outcome to the person
assigning values. Also, the mix and weighing of attributes vary among outcomes.
When an action can lead to different outcomes (e.g., death, pain, financial loss),
relative values for the different outcomes must be calculated on a common scale.

Choosing a scale for outcomes is related to the initial stages of decision
analysis when the problem was structured and a perspective defined. The options included as decision alternatives determine what outcomes must be assessed and valued. The viewpoint of the analysis influences how outcomes are
ranked and valued. For instance, an individual's utility for a health outcome may
be based on a scale of length and quality of that person's life. From a community's perspective, utility may be based on a scale of the number of lives saved
(i.e., deaths averted) as well as on quality of life.

Outcomes may be expressed in several ways, including "years of life expectancy," "number of lives saved," and "number of infections avoided." Outcomes may also be defined simply as costs or as the effectiveness of an intervention. Often in the health-policy area, health-status measures are used that
combine health information with other factors. Quality-adjusted life years is
a commonly used measure that combines qualitative and quantitative aspects
of outcomes. For a further discussion of quality-adjusted life years see chapter 9.

Averaging-Out-and-Folding-Back

Expected utility or *expected value* is a way of expressing in numbers which decision option would provide the highest value, cost, or other unit of measurement.
When outcomes are expressed as utilities, by definition, the decision option with
the highest expected utility *should* be preferred. Other decision rules apply when
outcomes are measured in other terms. See chapters 7, 8, and 9.

After all of the possible outcomes are quantified, expected utilities or expected values for each strategy can be calculated. The expected utility or expected value is the sum of the products of the estimates of the probability of

events and their outcomes. Mathematically, the expected utility or expected value for a chance node is calculated in two steps:

Step 1: The value of the outcome for each branch is multiplied by its respective probability.

Step 2: At each chance node, the products for the entire branch (calculated in Step 1) are summed (see Figure 3.5).

Expected utilities or expected values are first calculated for each branch of a decision tree at chance nodes, and then for each branch of a decision tree at decision nodes moving from the right side of the tree to the left. The process called *averaging-out-and-folding-back* is described below.

Beginning with the outcomes on the right, the value of the outcome at each terminal node is multiplied by the probability of that event's occurring. On branches of a chance node, products for each terminal node are summed. This is the expected value of the chance node. For example, calculate the expected value of the chance node at the top, far right branch of the vaccinate option in the tree in Figure 3.5. First, each of the three outcomes is multiplied by its respective probability of occurring:

Complete recovery	$8 \times 0.95 = 7.6$
Recovery but permanent disability	$5 \times 0.04 = 0.2$
Death	$0 \times 0.01 = 0$

Then, the values are summed to obtain the expected value of the chance node:

$$7.6 + 0.2 + 0 = 7.8$$

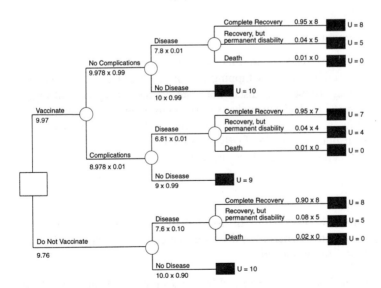

Figure 3.5 Expected values of outcomes in a decision tree with two options.

The process of averaging-out-and-folding-back continues to work toward the left side of the decision tree. (See Figure 3.5 for a decision tree with calculations completed.) In this part of the decision-analysis process, computerized decision-making programs can speed the straightforward but sometimes tedious mathematics needed to calculate the results of averaging-out-and-folding-back.

Although the decision tree presented in Figure 3.5 contains only one decision node (the root node), decision trees sometimes contain more than one decision node. When a decision tree contains additional decision nodes in addition to a root node, only the branch with the product of the highest numerical value is folded back. Branches with products of lower numerical value are "pruned" from the tree. This process is repeated from right to left until the initial decision point or root node is reached.

In cost-effectiveness analysis and cost-utility analysis, the process of averaging-out-and-folding-back is performed twice. The process is first completed using costs that occur on the path to the outcome at the terminal node. The second computation is done for effectiveness data as the measure of the outcome (e.g., cases prevented, quality-adjusted life years saved). The results of the two calculations are then combined in summary ratios described in chapters 8 and 9.

After the steps described above are completed, numerical results are available for the decision options at the initial decision node. Although performing the decision-tree calculations completes the initial process of the decision analysis, it is not the end of the decision-making process. The mathematical results need to be interpreted, and necessary adjustments must be made. Sensitivity analyses must also be done to evaluate the robustness of the expected-utility or expected-value calculations. Sensitivity analyses are described in detail below.

Harnessing Uncertainty

At this point, it is reasonable to wonder how this process compares to other decision-making methods such as flipping a coin or deciding on the basis of intuition. There may also be some discomfort with decision-analysis results that are based on estimates. If decision analyses were not used, however, there would still be uncertainty in the decision-making process. When decision analysis is used, the areas of uncertainty are clearly identified. It is useful to know with clarity what is uncertain, rather than subsuming the uncertainty into intuition.

Sensitivity Analysis
One way to harness the uncertainty of decision trees is to perform sensitivity analyses. With a sensitivity analysis, a decision tree can be mathematically manipulated to answer these questions:

- If the numerical estimate of a probability or an outcome is changed, how does expected utility or expected value change?

- How much would an estimate have to change to produce a different result, i.e., a higher expected value for another option?
- What value would a variable have to be for two strategies to have equal expected utility or expected value? (threshold analysis)
- What happens to the results of the model if "best-case scenario" estimates are used? If "worst-case" estimates are used?

For example, assume that in the decision analysis for vaccination, the probability estimate of 0.04 for recovery-but-permanent-disability following disease is based on an estimate from a panel of experts. The expert estimates might range from 0.005 to 0.10. A sensitivity analysis can be performed by recalculating with a value of 0.005 and then by recalculating with a value of 0.10. If one decision option continues to be preferable (because the expected utility is higher) no matter which estimate is used in the calculation, the decision maker should feel more comfortable with the process, since the uncertain estimate would not change the interpretation of the results of the decision tree.

A sensitivity analysis can be done by varying one parameter in a decision tree or by simultaneously varying two or more probability or utility estimates. When one value is changed (a one-way sensitivity analysis), the decision maker can see the effect of one variable on the entire decision tree. When several values are changed simultaneously in a multiway sensitivity analysis, the decision maker can examine the relationships among the various estimates used in the decision-tree calculations. Several types of sensitivity analyses are described below.

Threshold Analysis
A threshold analysis is a kind of sensitivity analysis that calculates the values of the point at which one should make a different decision, i.e., the expected-values or expected-utilities of two decision nodes are equivalent. With threshold analysis, one can determine how much a probability or outcome value would have to change for the decision tree to yield a sufficiently different value so a different decision option should be chosen. Again, threshold analyses can help the decision maker decide whether the uncertainty of estimates is large enough to question the interpretation of a decision analysis or whether there is enough confidence in the estimates to be comfortable with the decision.

For example, in the decision tree in Figure 3.5, the vaccination option has the highest expected value. This vaccine has a relatively low rate of complications. Suppose new clinical trials revealed that the complication rate was much higher. The decision analyst may ask at what complications rate would the expected value of the vaccination option be equal to the no vaccination option. A threshold analysis performed on the probability for complications following vaccination shows that the complication rate would have to rise to 22% before the vaccination option would no longer be the preferred strategy.

Threshold analysis can also be used to plan strategies for intervention programs. For example, in a screening program, an initial screen-all strategy might be preferred in a population with a certain prevalence of disease. Over time, as the prevalence of a disease has responded to screening and intervention, a selective-screening strategy may be more effective. Threshold analysis can help pinpoint the prevalence at which one strategy becomes more effective than another.

Threshold analysis has also been used to evaluate such cost factors as pricing schedules for pharmaceuticals. Threshold analysis can determine at what price a drug must be obtainable in order for a prevention intervention to be cost-effective on a large scale.

Monte Carlo Analysis
Monte Carlo analysis is a mathematically sophisticated sensitivity analysis based on the distributions of variables used in a decision tree. The two types of Monte Carlo analyses are called: *first order* and *second order*.

First Order. When a computer model decision tree is used, a first-order Monte Carlo analysis might run 10,000 hypothetical people through the tree, allowing the computer program to make selections randomly at each chance node. The results of the 10,000 hypothetical cases would be accumulated, and a distribution of the results would be generated by the computer. This distribution would provide some idea of the measure of central tendency and the variance of the results given the assumed, prespecified distribution of parameter values.

Second order. Again, when a computer model decision tree is used, a second-order Monte Carlo analysis might run a decision program 10,000 times. Rather than using a single estimate for a probability or a utility, a normal (or other) distribution would be designated. The computer would randomly select one of the values in the designated distribution for each of the 10,000 cases run through the decision model. The statistical results of the run of 10,000 hypothetical cases would provide information for further analysis and interpretation. For a given structure and set of parameter values, this distribution of results gives a measure of central tendency and variance of the results which could be expected across members of a cohort.

The information about the distribution of results obtained from either type of Monte Carlo analysis is very useful for understanding the robustness of the results to changes in parameter values and for estimating the range of results that cohort members might experience. Given the power of today's decision-analysis programs and of personal computers, the effort required to run Monte Carlo analysis is minimal.

Best- and Worst-Case Scenarios
In this kind of sensitivity analysis, the decision-tree model can be analyzed using low- or high-range estimates of variables that favor one option and can be reanalyzed using estimates that favor another option. If a decision is unchanged at extreme levels, the decision maker may gain confidence in the decision generated by the model.

COMMON CRITICISMS OF DECISION ANALYSIS

The previous sections have explained the process of decision analysis. Although decision analysis can be a useful tool in decision making, it cannot replace the human expertise and judgment required to make good decisions. To address some concerns that frequently arise, Weinstein, in his 1979 publication, *Sounding board, a decision analysis—a look at the chief complaints,* identified some common criticisms of decision analysis, together with some common responses.[9]

"Decision analysis takes too much time." Decision analysis does take time, but only a few decisions merit a full-blown decision analysis. Sometimes just structuring a problem clarifies the issues enough to allow a reasonable decision to be made.

"This is spurious quantification based on too many estimates and guesses." Uncertainty in decision making remains even if no decision analysis is performed. Decision analysis can help the process of sorting out what kinds of guesses are being used, regardless of what decision technique is used. In the process of decision analysis, decision makers can come to agreement on the question, the need for more information or research, and the probability and valuation of outcomes. By using experts to estimate probability and sensitivity analyses to interpret results, some of the uncertainty of decision analysis can be harnessed.

"Decisions should not be based on numbers. It is dehumanizing." Decision analysis recognizes that people value outcomes differently. Because expected utility includes not only probability but also desirability of outcomes in terms of human values, the process is responsive to the human side of making decisions.

"Computers will make all the decisions. Decision analysis takes the art out of judgment." The decision-analysis process is not automatic. The process requires expertise to lay out the trees. The analyst must be highly selective in structuring problems—deciding what options to choose, what outcomes to include, and what estimates are reasonable. A decision analysis can have a faulty result if a decision tree fails to include critical components. In addition to technology, the process of decision analysis also requires wisdom, skill, and knowledge. Ideally, decision analysis is done by a decision team that includes program-area experts, a decision expert, and a computer technician skilled in decision-tree programs. Decision analysis requires a change in thinking about how decisions are made. Using the techniques of decision analysis, the decision process is open to examination and vulnerable to criticism. The decision maker's values are apparent in terms of how a decision tree is structured and how outcomes are valued. Although this process helps to organize and clarify the decision-making process, it may also complicate the way decisions are made.

BENEFITS OF USING DECISION ANALYSIS IN PUBLIC HEALTH

In public health, decision analysis can benefit decision makers in several ways.

Explicitness

Unlike intuitive decision making, the decision-analysis process requires that options be clearly stated, consequences be clearly identified, and uncertainties be recognized. Decision rules may also be made explicit.

Comprehensiveness

When making a decision by intuition, a person is able to consider simultaneously only a limited number of options and to process a limited amount of information. Because the analysis process scrutinizes each part of a decision model for alternatives and outcomes, the process becomes more comprehensive than intuitive decision making can be.

Improvement of Communications

To one expert, the word *rarely* may mean a 1% chance; to another, it may mean a 10% chance. The process of decision analysis allows decision makers to understand and convey information clearly about aspects of a problem. With the use of formal decision analysis, it is also easy to document and justify the choices made. The decision-analysis process is also an excellent way to train others to make decisions.

Relief of Some Decision-Making Stress

Many people are uncomfortable about making decisions—especially complex decisions with far-reaching consequences. The logical, rational process of decision analysis lends structure, organization, and reason to a difficult process. Under pressure, decision making may become even more stressful. Decision analysis can assist in the formulation of rules for making decisions that can be used in a wide variety of settings.

Decision Analysis Encourages Focus

The process encourages decision makers to focus on truly important issues rather than on issues that merely seem to be important. Structuring a problem and conducting sensitivity analyses can clarify the significant issues involved in a decision.

In the Long Run, Expected-Utility Analysis Should Maximize Utility

Although the process may not confirm an intuitive decision, the process should result in optimizing choices. Decision analysis is, however, just one input into an array of factors and activities that influence decisions—including legal, political, distributional, financial, and ethical concerns.

CONCLUSION

This chapter has described how decision analysis can be used in the decision-making process and has presented an overview of decision analysis. Next, chapter 4 focuses on parameters most frequently found in prevention-effectiveness models. Readers are reminded that Appendix C and Appendix D contain self-study cases in decision analysis. These case studies illustrate and expand the concepts contained in chapter 3. Also, for a listing of decision-analysis software, see Appendix B.

CHECKLIST FOR EVALUATING A DECISION ANALYSIS

1. What is the question being addressed?
2. Is this question important?
3. Does the analysis take the societal perspective? If not, why not?
4. Are the options clearly identified?
5. Are the options appropriate? Are they realistic?
6. Have all reasonable options been considered?
7. What is the time horizon?
8. Does the decision tree flow in proper logical and chronological sequence?
9. Are the events at each chance node mutually exclusive and exhaustive?
10. Are any events included twice?
11. How have probabilities been determined?
12. What method is used to estimate utilities/costs/outcomes?
13. Is an appropriate scale used to estimate utilities/costs/outcomes?
14. What software is used to perform the mathematical calculations?
15. What sensitivity analyses are performed?
16. What are the threshold values for critical elements?
17. What other factors are to be considered in the decision-making process?

REFERENCES

1. Bottom WP, Bontempo RN, Holtgrave DR. Experts, novices, and the St. Petersburg Paradox: is one solution enough? *J Behav Decision Making* 1989;2:139–47.
2. von Neumann J, Morgenstern O. *Theory of games and economic behavior.* Princeton: Princeton University Press, 1947.
3. Schlaifer R. *Probability and statistics for business decisions: an introduction to managerial economics under uncertainty.* New York: McGraw-Hill, 1959.
4. Howard RA. *Decision analysis: applied decision theory.* In Hertz DB, Melese J (eds).

Proceedings of the Fourth International Conference on Operational Research. New York: Wiley-Interscience, 1966:55–71.
5. Ledley RS, Lusted LB. Reasoning foundations of medical diagnosis: symbolic logic, probability, and value theory aid our understanding of how physicians reason. *Science* 1959;130:819–24.
6. Henschke UK, Flehinger BJ. Decision theory in cancer therapy. *Cancer* 1967;20:1819–26.
7. Boadway RW, Bruce N. *Welfare economics*. New York: Basil Blackwell, 1990.
8. Yates JF. *Risk taking behavior*. New York: John Wiley and Sons, 1992.
9. Weinstein M. Sounding board, a decision analysis—a look at the chief complaints. *N Engl J Med* 1979;300:556–60.

BIBLIOGRAPHY

Theory of Decision Making
Arkes HR, Hammond KR (eds). *Judgment and decision making*. New York: Cambridge University Press, 1986.
Baron J. *Thinking and deciding*. New York: Cambridge University Press, 1988.
Bazerman MH. *Judgment in managerial decision making*, 2nd ed. New York: John Wiley and Sons, 1990.
Bottom WP, Bontempo RN, Holtgrave DR. Experts, novices, and the St. Petersburg Paradox: is one solution enough? *J Behav Decision Making* 1989;2:139–47.
Carroll JS, Johnson EJ. *Decision research: a field guide*. Newbury Park, CA: Sage, 1990.
Dawes RM. *Rational choice in an uncertain world*. New York: Harcourt Brace Jovanovich, 1988.
Dowie J, Elstein A (eds). *Professional judgment: a reader in clinical decision making*. New York: Cambridge University Press, 1988.
Hogarth R. *Judgment and choice*, 2nd ed. New York: John Wiley and Sons, 1987.
Kahneman D, Slovic P, Tversky A. *Judgment under uncertainty: heuristics and biases*. New York: Cambridge University Press, 1982.
Montgomery H, Svenson O (eds). *Process and structure in human decision making*. New York: John Wiley and Sons, 1989.
Russo JE, Schoemaker PJH. *Decision traps*. New York: Simon and Schuster, 1989.
Schwartz S, Griffin T. *Medical thinking*. New York: Springer-Verlag, 1986.
von Neumann J, Morgenstern O. *Theory of games and economic behavior*. Princeton: Princeton University Press, 1947.
Yates JF. *Judgment and decision making*. Englewood Cliffs, NJ: Prentice-Hall, 1990.
Yates JF. *Risk taking behavior*. New York: John Wiley and Sons, 1992.

Applied Decision Analysis
Bell DE, Raiffa H, Tversky A. *Decision making: descriptive, normative and prescriptive interactions*. New York: Cambridge University Press, 1988.
Gardenfors P, Sahlin N. *Decision, probability and utility*. New York: Cambridge University Press, 1988.
Keeney RL. *Decisions with multiple objectives: preferences and value trade-offs*. New York: John Wiley and Sons, 1976.
Sox, HC, Blatt MA, Higgins MC, Marton KI. *Medical decision making*. Stoneham, MA: Butterworth, 1988.

von Winterfeldt D, Edwards W. *Decision analysis and behavioral research.* New York: Cambridge University Press, 1986.
Watson SR, Buede D. *Decision synthesis.* New York: Cambridge University Press, 1987.
Weinstein M. Sounding board, a decision analysis—a look at the chief complaints. *N Engl J Med* 1979;300:556–60.

4

Decision Analysis for Public Health

STEVEN M. TEUTSCH
ANNE C. HADDIX

In public health decision making, characteristics of population cohorts or individuals influence expected outcome values for decision analyses. The probabilities used for screening characteristics and intervention effectiveness in a decision-tree model should reflect the population to which the model is applied. This chapter discusses the epidemiologic considerations of selecting decision alternatives to include in a decision tree and of determining the probability and outcome values to attach to them.

Because direct evidence of effectiveness is not usually available, estimating probabilities for a prevention-effectiveness analysis is important and must be done carefully. This chapter describes methods for estimating probabilities and includes several public health–related examples.

DETERMINING OPTIONS AT CHANCE NODES

As described in chapter 3, a decision tree comprises a series of branches that arise at nodes. Decision nodes generally include the major options or decisions that need to be made. For example, one might compare two decision options:

Option A: Cholesterol screening for young adults, followed by diet or drug therapy for those who have hypercholesterolemia.

Option B: No screening, but a recommendation that all young adults eat a "healthful" diet.

The options at this node are possible decision choices; that is, a decision maker may choose Option A or Option B.

Chance nodes, in contrast, represent events that occur as a consequence of a decision but over which one has *no control.* If Option A is selected, some of the young adults who receive treatment may experience side effects from drug therapy. The side effects are represented on a decision-tree model at a chance node rather than at a decision node because the side effects are a matter of chance—not something elected by the decision maker.

The branches at each chance node include the set of mutually exclusive and exhaustive events for which there is a probability of occurrence. Figure 4.1 illustrates a possible decision-tree model for the cholesterol screening example described above. In the example given above, for Option A (screening), one would need to consider the following questions:

- How likely are members of the young adult population to participate in a blood-cholesterol screening program?
- What are the sensitivity and specificity of the screening test (or tests, if follow-up testing is indicated)?
- What is the expected rate of compliance with diet therapy?
- What is the success of cholesterol reduction with diet counseling?
- If drug therapy is prescribed, what is the expected compliance with drug therapy?
- What are the side effects of the drugs?
- What is the success of drug therapy in cholesterol reduction and clinical outcome, such as evidence for reduction in coronary artery disease?

In a typical screening and treatment model such as that shown in Figure 4.1, chance nodes would represent the likelihood of involvement in screening, compliance, side effects, and outcomes. The decision-tree model should be structured in a logical, usually time-ordered, sequence. The variables in the tree should reflect factors relevant to the population being considered and to the method of intervention being considered. In an economic analysis, in addition to determining the probability of the occurrence of each event, one must also determine costs that accrue along each branch and the value of the outcomes identified at the terminal node for each branch. Costs and outcome values are discussed in subsequent chapters.

The following sections discuss the determination of the probabilities of the events within the structure of the tree, i.e., the probabilities that the branches will occur. They describe the types of variables most frequently found in decision trees for prevention interventions. Although many decision trees are structured in a similar style, the decision tree for each problem is unique; other variables in addition to those described below may need to be included in a model.

POPULATION CHARACTERISTICS

The probability and outcome measures selected for each decision tree must be suitable for the population the model is intended to represent. A decision tree may be used to calculate the expected outcomes of alternate prevention strategies for an individual or for a *cohort* of individuals. Calculating expected-outcome values for a heterogeneous cohort involves an additional step. For a

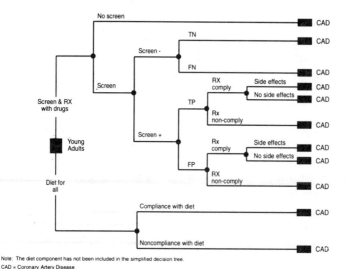

Note: The diet component has not been included in the simplified decision tree.
CAD = Coronary Artery Disease

Figure 4.1 A simplified decision tree for cholesterol screening and treatment among young adults.

heterogeneous cohort, the expected-outcome values for various groups that constitute the cohort are first determined separately and then are combined into a single expected outcome for the entire cohort.

The way a decision model is constructed for a heterogeneous cohort is also important. The *same* cohort must be used for each branch emanating from the *decision node*. Once the cohort reaches a chance node in the tree, the cohort can be divided appropriately. For example, if a heterogeneous cohort comprises a group of males and females ages 45–60 years, the entire and identical mixed-gender group will be used as the cohort for each branch at the initial decision node. It is not permissible to have the male group follow one decision path from the decision node while the females follow another. At chance nodes, however, the cohort group might be split to reflect differences. In the mixed-gender group above, treatment strategies may be different for men and women; thus, the subsequent branches of the decision tree would reflect the steps each subgroup follows through the model.

Often the first chance node on a decision branch incorporates the characteristics of the population relevant to the prevention problem. The characteristics of the relevant population may be demographic (often used to delineate target groups), may be related to the prevalence of a disease or injury, or may be socio/behavioral. Characteristics of a population are important in three instances.

In the first case, target groups may be different for the options being considered. Indeed, a particular group may be identified as a target group on the basis of its behavioral risk factors or the prevalence of disease for that group. The case study in Appendix D illustrates this point. In this case study, two strategies are analyzed in a hypothetical decision analysis for Disease XYZ involving the U. S. population as the cohort:

Option A: Only the segment of the population with behavioral characteristics associated with increased risk of the disease, the "high-risk" group, would be vaccinated.

Option B: The entire population would be targeted for vaccination.

In this example, the first chance node represented the probability that a member of the population was or was not in the high-risk group. Thus, the characteristics of the population being considered were directly related to the strategy selected.

Second, optional interventions may affect different population groups differently. For example, in a recent analysis of alternate strategies to increase folic acid intake of women of child-bearing age to reduce the incidence of neural tube birth defects,[1] three strategies were considered: (1) nutritional counseling, (2) fortification of grain products, and (3) distribution of vitamin supplements. The cohort of interest was the U. S. female population 15–45 years of age. Although folic acid is known to prevent neural tube defects among children, the consumption of folic acid may also mask pernicious anemia among older people. Thus although the target group for each folic-acid intervention strategy was the same (women of child-bearing age), the costs and the adverse effects of the alternate strategies were distributed differently throughout the remainder of the population. Therefore, the first node after the decision was the "population node," which separated the target group (women of child-bearing age) from the rest of the population over 15 years of age. The two probabilities at this node are that a member of the cohort is a female of child-bearing age (p), and the probability that a member is not in that group ($1 - p$).

The third instance in which characteristics of population are important in decision analysis is when probabilities encountered later in the process depend on the characteristics of the population. This point is illustrated by the example presented in Figure 4.1. In this model, variables conditional on population characteristics are likely to be (1) the prevalence of hypercholesterolemia, (2) compliance with diet therapy in the absence of screening, (3) compliance with diet after screening positive, and (4) the risk of coronary artery disease. To evaluate the variables, one needs to know the probabilities for each factor for young adults, because young adults have been defined as the target group. Data derived from information on middle-aged males should not be used unless there is reason to believe that it is applicable to the younger population and unless there is no more relevant information available.

Many public health decision analyses target specific populations. For example, a study examining the cost-effectiveness of a national screening program for cystic fibrosis (CF) in Israel targeted couples where both persons were of Ashkenazi origin—a risk factor carrying the CF gene—to identify carriers.[2] Another decision analysis examined the costs and benefits of implementing a mental status screening program for older drivers.[3] Older drivers were selected as the target population because (1) older drivers have higher rates of motor vehicle collisions; (2) there is concern that cognitive impairment, especially dementia, affects driving skills; and (3) there is a higher prevalence of dementia in the elderly. A third example of decision analyses targeting specific populations is two studies which examine the cost-effectiveness of vaccinating for hepatitis B vaccine. One study targets infants for vaccination.[4] The second examines the cost-effectiveness of two target populations: infants and adolescents.[5]

The more precisely demographic and socioeconomic characteristics can be specified, the more precisely the results can be determined. The trade-off, however, is that as the population is specified with more precision, it may become more difficult to obtain applicable data for the tightly defined group. Nonetheless, it is important that the relevant population be specified and that the most appropriate data be obtained. When data are not available and it is not feasible to conduct a study to determine the values, it may be possible to use estimates derived from other populations. The range of plausible estimates should then be subjected to sensitivity analyses (see chapter 3). If the sensitivity analyses show that small changes in the value of a variable have a substantial effect on the results of the analysis, more precise estimates are required to reduce the uncertainty of the decision model. However, if the sensitivity analyses show that changes in the variable have no effect on the results of the analysis over the range of plausible estimates, the analyst may decide that the estimated value is acceptable for the model.

SCREENING PARAMETERS

Many trees begin with the assumption that there is a population of people with and without a condition or of persons who may or may not benefit from some type of intervention. Decision trees are usually divided into two branches at this point. Each population is then subjected to alternate interventions. For clinical interventions, one of the first steps may be to triage the population into subgroups of persons who should and should not receive an intervention. A common way to do this is with a screening test to determine persons at highest risk. Examples of decision analyses for screening tests include screening men over 30 years of age for hereditary hemochromatosis[6] and ophthalmoscopic examination for detecting diabetic retinopathy.[7]

For any screening test, only part of the population will be screened, because the intervention is already present in the community or because individuals are not screened for some reason. This raises issues of whether those who are not screened differ in some way from those who are. In some instances, higher-risk individuals may present for screening (e.g., when a person has a family history of the health problem in question), whereas in other situations, high-risk individuals may not present for screening (e.g., when they have poor access to or cannot afford a screening test). Estimates are needed of the rates of compliance with screening and any differential risk patterns that might exist among those who are not screened.

The screening test itself is used to identify persons who should have the intervention in question. The screening test is used to identify "true positives," i.e., true cases, and "true negatives"; however, all screening tests also have "false positives" and "false negatives." Persons in all four of these groups must be identified as separate branches on the decision tree, since risks, costs, and benefits will accrue differently to each group.

In the simplest case, the true-positives group will be subjected to the intervention and its risks, but will also accrue its benefits. The false-positives group will also be subjected to the intervention—its costs and its risks—but since they do not have the condition (for which screening is being conducted), they will not receive any benefits from the intervention. Similarly, the true-negatives group will not receive the intervention but presumably will have a lower rate of the outcome being examined. However, the false-negative group will not receive the intervention and will have a comparable rate of outcome to that for any other untreated group of people with the health problem.

Information on the sensitivity and specificity of the screening test are generally characteristic of the test itself. These probabilities are added to the tree, the sensitivity to the "cases" branch to identify the true positives and false negatives; and the specificity to the noncases as the true negatives and false positives. Thus the proportion of individuals in each of the four categories (TN, FN, TP, FP) is a function of the sensitivity and specificity of the laboratory test as well as of the underlying prevalence of the condition for which screening is conducted. The same general set of principles applies when screening methods other than laboratory tests are used, e.g., questionnaires, physical examination, or some other method of identifying individuals or populations at risk. An example of the latter is a cost-effectiveness analysis of selected versus universal screening of women in STD clinics for *Chlamydia trachomatis*.[8] The selected screening option uses a combination of behavioral risk factors and physical signs to determine if treatment is warranted.

Another factor that may need to be added to a tree is the rate at which patients are followed up in order to obtain test results. In counseling and testing for HIV infection, for instance, many clients do not return to a clinic to obtain test results. Because testing is anonymous, clients who do not return cannot be traced.

LINKING RISK FACTORS TO HEALTH PROBLEMS

Screening programs may be designed to identify risk factors. For example, pregnant women who have positive results in screening for alcohol use may be at risk of giving birth to a child with fetal alcohol syndrome. The next step in the model is to assess the likelihood of developing a given health outcome following exposure to that risk factor. In other models, the screening step may not be needed. However, linking risk factors to the health problem is still a critical step.

Risk can be established on the basis of the incidence for a population with a given set of characteristics. This information can be gleaned from population-based studies. If incidence is known for some groups but not others, it can be calculated using relative risks or risk ratios to compare the group with the known incidence to groups with an unknown level of risk.

DETERMINING THE IMPACT OF AN INTERVENTION

When an intervention strategy has been tested in community-based settings, the impact should be measured in terms of the reduction in the incidence of a specific outcome. In an entire population, this reduction, the prevented fraction (see Appendix J), may be expressed as an absolute or as a percentage reduction in incidence. The incidence for each risk group (e.g., persons who have and have not been subjected to an intervention) can be used in the model to determine the risk of each health outcome.

Often, explicit studies demonstrating the impact of an intervention have not been conducted. It is necessary to estimate the *potential* effect of an intervention. This can be done if one knows the relative risk of the factor being addressed, e.g., the relative risk of myocardial infarction for persons with hypercholesterolemia. The relative risk, population prevalence of the risk factor, and incidence of the health outcome are used to determine the attributable risk, or the incidence of a health outcome which can be attributed to a risk factor (see Appendix J). The attributable risk measures the amount of the health problem that could have been prevented if the risk factor had never existed. This represents the maximum benefit that a prevention program could achieve. In decision models, this maximum limit needs to be adjusted for compliance, penetration of the intervention, and risk that was incurred before the intervention was implemented.

INTERVENTION EFFECTIVENESS

The effectiveness of the intervention is the product of its efficacy, compliance, and penetration. When data are directly available on effectiveness from a suitable community-based study, these three factors may already be included in an overall summary measure. If data are not available in this form, the analyst may incorporate these variables into a model as separate entities. Also, if efficacy, compliance, and penetration are constant for each group that receives the intervention, the factors can be combined into a single step for the sake of simplicity.

In many instances, data on efficacy may be available, e.g., from randomized control clinical trials. However, data on efficacy provide information on the impact of an intervention in ideal populations under ideal circumstances. This level of success can rarely be achieved in a routine clinical or community setting. In typical community settings, an intervention may not reach all subjects who might benefit (penetration). Because the efficacy and penetration are probably higher in ideal circumstances than they are in community settings, efficacy and penetration must be factored into a prevention-effectiveness model.

By the same token, all those who initially participate may not continue to comply with an intervention, and compliance, too, must be incorporated into the model. When compliance varies by group, it should be included as a separate step. Compliance may vary, e.g., among groups with different perceived levels of risk. Persons with very high levels of blood cholesterol may be more compliant with dietary recommendations than those with moderately high levels of blood cholesterol; and those with moderately high levels may, in turn, be more compliant than a population with normal cholesterol levels or than a group that has not been tested for cholesterol.

Estimates of penetration and compliance should be obtained from the data on a comparable population involved with the same intervention, when possible. When this information is not available, data from similar interventions might be used and tested using a range of possible values by using sensitivity analyses.

An example of a decision analysis that incorporated efficacy and compliance variables for two alternative drug therapies was a cost-effectiveness analysis of single-dose azithromycin versus multidose doxycycline for the treatment of *Chlamydia trachomatis* in women.[9] In this study, the two therapies were equally efficacious. The decision result hinged on the differences in compliance rates for the two drugs.

In addition to efficacy, compliance, and penetration, other factors must also be considered. Most interventions have some undesirable effects associated with them, and these, too, need to be incorporated into the model. Side effects of drugs are readily identified; side effects of screening programs may not be as easily discernible, but may also cause harm. Mammography screening, for example, may lead to such side effects as anxiety on the part of the client because of a positive test result, unnecessary biopsies, and complications following biopsies. These risks may be incorporated as separate branches in the model. The frequency of the risk for side effects is incorporated at the probability node, but the value of these risks is incorporated into the outcome node in a decision analysis.

One example of a decision analysis that incorporated side effects into the decision model is a cost-effectiveness analysis of empiric treatment of tick bites to prevent Lyme disease.[10] Because an empiric treatment strategy results in the treatment of some patients who do not have the disease, major and minor antibiotic complications were explicitly included as health outcomes in addition to the cases of Lyme disease prevented. The costs of the side effects were included as additional cost parameters.

SOURCES OF ESTIMATES OF THE PROBABILITIES

Most decision models use information synthesized from a variety of studies. Often studies have not been performed to provide the information needed for estimating all the variables in the model. Where, then, can one get the information needed? A good starting point is a list of the variables in the model, followed by consideration of which of the following sources might be appropriate for obtaining an estimate.

Literature

A search of the literature may be used to determine probability values. Some of the variables are biologic phenomena that would be expected to be comparable in different populations, e.g., the risk of developing coronary artery disease for white males who have hypercholesterolemia and are in specific age groups should be the same regardless of place of residence. Other variables may be highly context-dependent, e.g., compliance rates with different intensity of intervention and follow up.

When multiple values are found, the most reliable estimate can be determined by considering the scientific validity of available studies and by examining the similarity of the population in the published study to the population being considered. Methods for evaluating published studies might include a *meta-analysis*, in which multiple studies with disparate results have been systematically combined (see Appendix K), or a variety of consensus or delphi techniques involving an expert panel.

Unpublished Studies

Data may be available from unpublished studies based on practical experience with the intervention in question or similar interventions. The probabilities for compliance and follow up may be obtained from community-based experience in public health programs. These probabilities are likely to vary substantially from those of carefully controlled efficacy studies and may actually be more appropriate for decision analyses for public programs. The quality of the data should be carefully considered.

Expert Opinion

When no objective information is available, expert opinion may be sought. For example, the literature may not have data on the typical follow-up evaluation of an individual who has a positive screening-test result. A group of practicing clinicians with expertise in diagnosing and treating persons for this condition could be surveyed to determine the treatment procedures they typically use. Experts may also provide their opinion regarding likely probabilities for other factors; however, these estimates may be based on populations of patients seen by these particular experts—a population which may differ substantially from a general population. In such a situation, sensitivity analyses with wide intervals may be necessary. Details on specialized procedures, such as characteristics of laboratory tests, are often available from experts.

National Surveys

Data may be available from proprietary data bases such as IMS's *National Disease and Therapeutic Index,* and surveillance systems such as the Consumer Product Safety Commission's NEISS or CDC's surveillance systems. Data bases include the National Center for Health Statistics' Health and Nutrition Examination Survey, Hospital Discharge Survey, and Health Interview Survey. A description of several national surveys useful for prevention-effectiveness research is provided in Appendix E.

Limited Studies

When information is not readily available, some of the data may be secured from special studies. For example, compliance rates might be determined from a record review.

Estimates

When probabilities cannot be obtained, investigators may need to determine plausible values and use a broad range of estimates in sensitivity analyses. When sensitivity analyses find that conclusions are sensitive to plausible variable values, more precise estimates will be needed. Thus, sensitivity analyses can help to determine which variables in a model warrant more intensive investigation or further studies to obtain more precise estimates.

CONCLUSION

Analytic models should be constructed so as to describe explicitly all important steps in a decision. Probabilities for each of the variables in a decision model must be obtained. When estimates are not readily available from the published literature, expert opinion, or limited studies, plausible estimates can be used. Sensitivity analyses should always be performed to determine whether decisions would be altered over a plausible range for each variable. In such a case, research should be focused on the critical variables for which more precise estimates are needed.

REFERENCES

1. Kelly AE, Scanlon KS, Mulinare J, Helmick CG, Haddix AC. Cost-effectiveness of alternative strategies to prevent neural tube defects in *Cost-effectiveness in Health and Medicine,* Gold MR, Siegel JE, Russell LB, Weinstein MC (eds). New York: Oxford University Press, 1966.
2. Ginsberg G, Blau H, Kerem E, Springer C et al. Cost-benefit analysis of a national screening programme for cystic fibrosis in an Israeli population. *Health Economics* 1994;3:5–24.

3. Retchin SM, Hillner BE. The costs and benefits of a screening program to detect dementia in older drivers. *Med Decision Making* 1994;14(4):315–24.
4. Krahn M, Detsky AS. Should Canada and the United States universally vaccinate infants against Hepatitis B? A cost-effectiveness analysis. *Med Decision Making* 1993;13:4–20.
5. Bloom BS, Hillman AL, Fendrick AM, Schwartz JS. A reappraisal of Hepatitis B virus vaccination strategies using cost-effectiveness analysis. *Ann Intern Med* 1993;118:298–306.
6. Phatak PD, Guzman G, Woll JE, Robeson A, Phelps CE. Cost-effectivness of screening for hereditary hemochromatosis. *Arch Intern Med* 1994;154:769–76.
7. Dasbach EJ, Fryback DG, Newcomb PA et al. Cost effectiveness of strategies for detecting diabetic retinopathy. *Med Care* 1991;8:644–50.
8. Marrazzo JM, Celum CL, Fine D, DeLisle S, Mosure DJ, Handsfield HH. Cost-effectiveness of selective vs. universal screening for *Chlamydia trachomatis* infection in women attending family planning and STD clinics. Orfila J et al (ed). Chlamydial infections: Proceedings of the eighth international symposium on human chlamydial infections. Bologna: Societa Editrice Esculapio, 1994:63–66.
9. Haddix AC, Hillis SD, Kassler WJ. The cost-effectiveness of azithromycin for *Chlamydia trachomatis* infections in women. *J Sexually Transmitted Dis* 1995; 22:274–80.
10. Magid D, Schwartz B, Craft J, Schwartz JS. Prevention of Lyme disease after tick bites, a cost-effectiveness analysis. *N Engl J Med* 1992;327:534–39.

BIBLIOGRAPHY

Eddy DM, Hasselblad V, Schacter R. *Meta-analysis by the confidence profile method.* New York: Academic Press, 1992.
Elixhauser A (ed.). Health care cost-benefit and cost-effectiveness analysis (CBA/CEA) from 1979 to 1990: a bibliography. *Med Care* 1993;31: Suppl.
Hedges LV, Olkin I. *Statistical methods for meta-analysis.* San Diego: Academica Press, 1985.
Petitti DB. *Meta-analysis decision analysis and cost-effectiveness analysis.* New York: Oxford University Press, 1994.
Sox HC Jr, Blatt MA, Higgins MC, Marton KI. *Medical decision making.* Boston: Butterman-Heinemann, 1988.

5

Cost of an Intervention

ROBIN D. GORSKY
ANNE C. HADDIX
PHAEDRA A. SHAFFER

The cost of implementing a prevention strategy is an essential component of all prevention-effectiveness studies. This chapter discusses the collection and analysis of data needed to calculate the cost of a specific intervention or program. It covers the three components of the cost of an intervention: (1) program costs, (2) costs to participants, and (3) costs associated with side effects of the intervention. Further information on the estimation of intervention costs can be found in the literature.[1-6]

TYPES OF INTERVENTION COST STUDIES

The strategy for estimating costs of an intervention depends on whether the study is designed as a *retrospective* study, a *model* of prevention interventions, or a *prospective* study. We emphasize data collection for a prospective cost analysis in this chapter.

In a *retrospective study*, the researcher attempts to identify the program costs after the program has begun or been completed. Often no cost data have been collected for a program, or they are imprecise and incomplete. Some costs such as the cost of participating in the intervention (e.g., time and travel costs) may be impossible to estimate at this stage. When conducting a retrospective cost analysis, all relevant cost categories should be identified. Costs that are omitted from the study because of lack of data should be described explicitly. The presentation of the study should include a discussion of the possible effects caused by omitting costs in the analysis. Studies should also state explicitly any assumptions about cost estimates and should give results of sensitivity analyses on estimates of intervention costs.

Prevention-effectiveness models are studies designed to predict the most cost-effective strategy *before* a strategy is implemented. Intervention costs in prevention-effectiveness models are based on the projected costs of an intervention. Because actual cost data are not available and models are based on estimates, all assumptions regarding costs should be explicitly stated. Results of sensitivity analyses on estimates of intervention costs should be presented with the study results together with a discussion of the possible effect of using costs different from those of the model.

In a *prospective study*, consistent and reliable cost estimates may be obtained, since actual cost data can be collected while the intervention program is in effect. The researcher may decide in advance what cost information is needed for the study. Then complete and accurate cost data may be collected for the analysis. The following sections focus on collection of cost while an intervention is being delivered. The three main steps in determining costs of an intervention include: (1) developing a cost inventory, (2) collecting inventory costs, and (3) calculating total expected costs of an intervention.

DEVELOPING A COST INVENTORY

Determining the costs of an intervention is a complex and time-consuming task. For the sake of completeness, a good approach is to develop an inclusive inventory of all the costs necessary to implement the intervention. The costs to include in the inventory depend on the following:

1. Study perspective
2. Time period for collection of resource data
3. Unit of intervention
4. Other possible interventions being assessed
5. Availability of data

Once these factors are determined, an inventory can be created which identifies the resources required to provide the intervention.[7]

At this point it is useful to distinguish between two concepts of cost: *financial costs* and *economic costs*. The financial costs of an intervention are the money outlays for resources required to produce the intervention, e.g., salaries, rent, office supplies. The economic costs of an intervention are the opportunity costs of the resources used to implement the intervention, i.e., the value of the resources if those resources had been used for another productive purpose. Economic costs provide a more complete estimate of intervention costs than financial costs because they include *all* the resources used to implement a prevention strategy. Not only do economic costs include program expenditures, they also include program resources for which *no* money was spent, e.g., volunteer time, space in the local public health department, donated brochures.

In many circumstances the economic cost of a resource may differ from the financial cost. The classic example is the distinction between costs and charges for medical services. The economic cost, measured as the opportunity cost of the resources used to deliver the medical service, is often substantially different from the charge for the medical service, measured as the amount paid for the service. (Chapter 8 provides a more detailed discussion of the cost versus charge dilemma.) Because it is important to capture fully the value of the resources required for prevention-effectiveness studies, the economic costs of a program or intervention should be used.

Study Perspective

The selection of the study perspective helps determine which costs should be included. If the study takes a societal perspective, all cost categories will be relevant. However, if a health-care-provider perspective is to be used, costs for participants or patients may not be included. When conducting a study from multiple perspectives it is helpful to construct a table of intervention costs based upon the inventory list with columns for each perspective.

Time Period

During the delivery of an intervention, costs occur as clients are served. Three factors are important when selecting a time period over which to collect intervention costs: (1) the time period for the cost data collection must be contemporaneous with the time period for which clients are served; (2) the time period should be long enough to avoid any secular patterns, e.g., seasonal effects; and (3) the time period should be of sufficient length to capture program start-up and maintenance costs.

Several factors influence the selection of the time period for a study. First, it is important that the cost data are collected for the same time period for which clients are served. In some facilities, cost data may be available for a fiscal year, whereas the number of tests or persons participating in programs may be available by calendar year. The time period selected should allow matching of the cost data to client outcomes.

Second, selection of the time period depends upon whether seasonality or other time patterns affect either costs or client participation. A time period of less than 1 year may have bias in the result due to seasonal effects on participation and behavior. A 1-year time period is generally recommended. It is unwise to collect data for less than 1 year unless there is known to be no seasonal effect.

Time periods greater than 1 year may also be used; however, they require a decision about how to incorporate cost increases and changes in technology over time. Studies of interventions lasting longer than 1 year must also use discounting to account for the time value of resources expended in future years.[2] A longer time period may also be appropriate because of the duration of the intervention or the time lag between the start-up of the intervention and the effect it creates.

Finally, in addition to annual maintenance costs of the intervention, start-up costs should also be collected, since they must also be reflected in calculating the overall cost of an intervention. If the time period selected for study includes the start-up period for the intervention, an additional 1 year of cost data after the start-up period has ended should be included so the cost data reflect ongoing costs. Often, for multiyear programs with significant start-up costs, an annual program cost is calculated to allow the use of a 1-year time frame in the prevention-effectiveness study. Construction of an annual cost requires the annuitization of the program's capital resources that will not be exhausted during the lifetime of the program.

Intervention Unit

Results of cost analyses must be summarized in a usable form for integration into prevention-effectiveness analyses. Generally, results of cost analyses are expressed as a rate, i.e., cost per intervention unit. One of the most common intervention units is the person offered or beginning an intervention, e.g., cost per 10^n persons exposed to the intervention. To calculate the average cost per 10^n persons offered the intervention, the total cost for the specified time period is divided by total persons offered the intervention and multiplied by 10^n, to obtain the average cost per 10^n persons offered the intervention. For example, if Program A costs \$1,200,000 to serve 1,200 clients and Program B costs \$500,000 to serve 400 clients, the average cost per 100 clients is \$100,000 in Program A and \$125,000 in Program B.

Depending on the structure of the prevention-effectiveness study, more than one intervention rate may need to be estimated from the intervention cost analysis. Most frequently, the need for multiple intervention rates occurs with programs which have varying degrees of participant completion. For example, consider a routine childhood vaccination program in which only 60% of children participating in the program complete the three-dose series. Thirty percent receive two doses and 10% receive only one dose. The cost analysis for this study will be used to determine three intervention rates: (1) the cost per child receiving three doses; (2) the cost per child receiving two doses; and (3) the cost per child receiving only one dose.

This rate is also useful in determining the *net costs* of the alternative strategies in prevention-effectiveness studies because most health-outcome rates are also expressed as some number per 10^n persons. In prevention-effectiveness analyses the intervention costs are often compared to the costs that would be incurred if no intervention was offered. For example, assume the cost of immunizing 1,000 persons against a particular disease is \$25,000. (Assume the vaccine is 100% efficacious.) If the expected rate of disease in an unvaccinated population is 1 case per 1,000 persons and the cost of treating an infected person is \$25,000, then the cost in the absence of the immunization program would be \$25,000. Thus, the vaccine program would yield no net savings and provide no justification *on the basis of cost* to spend \$25,000 to immunize 1,000 persons.

When prevention-effectiveness studies examine multiple interventions, comparability may depend on the use of a common intervention rate, e.g., cost per member of birth cohort, cost per clinic patient. The conversion of program costs to either a marginal or average rate allows a comparison among several interventions of different sizes for the same health outcome.

The distinction between *average* and *marginal* costs is critical to producing a valid prevention-effectiveness study. The marginal cost of one intervention *cannot* be compared with the average cost of an alternative intervention. These two types of costs are defined and compared below.

An *average* cost is the total resource cost, including all support and overhead costs, divided by the total units of output,

$$average\ cost\ =\ TC\ /\ Q \tag{1}$$

where TC = total costs and Q = outputs.

A *marginal* cost is the resource costs associated with producing one *additional* unit of the same intervention. Marginal cost can be calculated by dividing the change in total costs that results from a marginal change in activity to the change in output obtained from one additional unit of the same intervention.

$$marginal\ costs\ =\ (TC'\ -\ TC)\ /\ (Q'\ -\ Q) \tag{2}$$

Because marginal costs are a function of the size of a public health program, the marginal cost per unit of output of an intervention can be greater than or less than the average cost per unit of output. When a marginal analysis of a program is conducted, it is important to consider whether the program is operating at its most efficient size. Because this is difficult to determine, prevention-effectiveness studies often implicitly assume that programs are operating at optimal efficiency. The relationship between average and marginal costs at different levels of output is illustrated in an example in Table 5.1.[8] In this example, the marginal cost is initially less than the average cost; however, as additional units are produced and additional fixed costs must be incurred to expand production, the marginal cost of an additional unit of output exceeds the average cost of that unit.

Other Interventions Being Assessed

Next, the number of resources on the inventory which need to be collected can be potentially reduced by determining disparities in the alternative interventions. Because collection of cost data is complex and time-consuming, limiting the costs needed to conduct an analysis may streamline a study while still providing the necessary information for decision making. Sometimes two very

Table 5.1 Total, Average, and Marginal Costs

No. of Units (Q)	Total Costs (TC)	Average Costs (AC)	Marginal Costs (MC)
20	4,000	200	
40	6,000	150	100
60	7,000	117	50
80	10,000	125	150
100	15,000	150	250

similar interventions differ, for example, only in the type of screening test or the drug used for therapy. In this kind of analysis, all costs except for the costs of tests and their associated administrative costs (if different for the two interventions) or the cost of the alternative medications can be excluded. The *marginal* cost of each intervention strategy rather than the *total* cost of the strategy is calculated when interventions are similar. However, if the interventions differ markedly in structure, it is usually necessary to determine the total cost of each intervention.

For the purpose of *comparing* more than one program in an economic analysis, *incremental* costs need to be defined. *Incremental* costs refer to the cost differences (additional costs) between two programs. Compared to average and marginal cost, *incremental cost* refers to the cost of producing one additional unit of output by each alternative intervention.

Availability of Data

The final step in developing a cost inventory before the data collection process begins is to determine whether the necessary data exist. As mentioned before, if data are not available, a decision will have to be made to exclude the cost or to estimate it based on assumptions drawn from other sources. Once these factors have all been determined, the final step is to list the resources or inputs to be collected.

COLLECTION OF INTERVENTION COSTS

Once the parameters of the cost analysis have been established, a cost inventory is developed. The cost inventory is a comprehensive list of all the resources required to carry out an intervention. Depending on the perspective of the analysis, this list will include (1) program costs, (2) costs to participants, and (3) costs associated with side effects of the intervention. Types of inputs that may appear in the cost inventory are:

- Personnel costs including the salary or hourly wages and fringe benefits. Personnel costs may include:
    - direct-provider time for each type of service or activity, by provider type
    - support staff
    - administrative staff
    - volunteers
- Supplies and materials associated with each type of service provided
- Laboratory costs for each service provided including tests and controls
- Drug costs
- Facilities, including rent and utilities
- Maintenance for facilities and equipment
- Equipment

- Transportation costs and travel expenses
- Educational materials
- Media expenses including production, airtime, and space
- Training costs
- Outside consultant services
- Evaluation costs
- Other direct costs of providing services, e.g., courier services, uniforms or badges, additional insurance or permits, and construction and maintenance of a computer data base
- Participant time and expenses

An example of a list of intervention costs for an HIV counseling program may be found in Table 5.2.[9]

Once the cost inventory has been completed, costs must be categorized in such a way that average and marginal costs can be calculated. The costs which are included in calculating the cost of an intervention fall into two categories: fixed and variable costs. *Fixed* costs are those whose total remains constant (within a relevant range) even though the volume of the activity may vary. Examples include rent, design and production of advertising media, and capital expenditures for equipment. *Variable* costs are those that respond proportion-

Table 5.2 A Resource Inventory for a Hypothetical 1-Year HIV Counseling Program

Resource	Unit	Cost/Unit
FIXED COSTS		
Personnel[a]		
Administrator	year	64,421.00
Clerical worker	year	14,375.00
Facilities		
Rent	month	1,485.00
Maintenance	month	240.00
Utilities	month	150.00
Phone	month	86.00
Supplies & Equipment		
Office supplies	month	450.00
Computer[b]	year	1,900.00
VARIABLE COSTS		
Personnel[a]		
Counselor	hour	22.44
Supplies & Misc.		
Client education materials	set	2.80
Travel	mile	0.28
Participant Costs[c]		
Travel	mile	0.28

[a] Includes benefits
[b] Annualized cost of capital equipment
[c] Productivity losses not included

ately to change in volume of activity. Examples of variable costs include test kits for human immunodeficiency virus (HIV), bicycle helmets, and condoms.

In determining the cost of an intervention, in the short run fixed costs do not change in response to the number of clients being served. Variable costs, in contrast, vary with the number of clients served. It is important to distinguish between fixed and variable costs so costs may be calculated correctly for the number of clients used in the analysis. Methods for calculating variable and fixed cost components of the cost of an intervention are described below. The next step in a cost analysis is collecting and analyzing the costs of the resources outlined in the cost inventory.

Program Costs

Prevention programs incur costs for implementation and maintenance. If resources are allocated for one intervention, they cannot be used for other interventions. Cost data for different programs may be used for decision making on the basis of alternative uses or the *opportunity cost* of public resources. This section describes the collection and analysis of types of costs frequently found in prevention programs.

Variable Costs

Provider Time. In interventions where providers deliver services, provider time can be determined through four methods: (1) direct observation of service durations; (2) random observations of provider activities (snapshots in time); (3) time diaries completed by providers; and (4) patient flow analysis using time forms that a client carries from provider to provider. The correct sample sizes for estimating provider times can be derived from the statistical and epidemiologic references cited below.

Direct observation of services is the most accurate method. However this method requires that each provider be followed by a trained observer who can differentiate among services and correctly record the start time and stop time of each service. Direct observation usually requires consent of the client. At least 25 and as many as 100 observations may be required to obtain a confident estimate of time durations.[4] To determine the number of observations needed, a histogram may be constructed. If the histogram shows symmetry and small variation, 25 observations may be sufficient; however, a distribution with the mean equal to the standard deviation would suggest that 100 observations are needed to correctly estimate provider time.

Random observation uses the analogy that the proportion of observations of a particular service equals the actual proportion of time spent providing a particular service. In this method, providers are assigned a code number. The analyst chooses provider numbers from a random number table and prepares a list. This list is used to find, at fixed intervals, a specific provider and to note the service being provided at the exact moment of observation. At least five observations of each service type must be obtained for the proportionality assumption to hold, based upon the multinomial distribution.[5]

Time diaries allow self-observation by providers to record service to clients.

Time diaries are generally kept on a sheet of paper carried by the provider for each day. The diary is divided into rows and columns. Rows represent new activities or services. Each row has a check-off list (columns) for the specific type of activity being performed, including personal time, and a large final column for comments or explanations. To construct a check-off list which minimizes the provider time required to complete the diary, a pilot observation of a usual day must be made.

When using the time diary, the provider notes the start time of each activity (one activity = one row) in the first column. Since all activities are included in this continuous stream of activities, only the activity start time is needed. The start time of the next activity is the end time of the previous one. At least 25 self-observations or diary entries of each activity are required.[5]

Patient flow analysis requires a time form that the client carries from provider to provider, beginning with the receptionist at the time the patient checks in for the program. Ideally this form includes a space to note the time the client arrives at a program, is seen by the first service provider, leaves the provider, sees subsequent providers, and finally leaves the program. Again, data from at least 25 clients for each type of service are needed for an accurate analysis of provider time.

The cost of provider time is calculated by multiplying the time spent by the cost for that time. The hourly rate of compensation for the service provider including the fringe benefits paid to that employee must be included. Employee fringe benefits are included as a cost of doing business and must be included in calculating the cost of an intervention. Information on salary and benefits can usually be obtained from the administrator or financial officer of the program.

Provider cost is determined for each provider type by using the following equation

$$\text{provider cost} = (\text{provider salary} + \text{benefits}) \times \text{duration of service} \times \text{number of services provided in time period} \tag{3}$$

Other Variable Costs. The costs of materials, supplies, tests, and other resources associated with particular services are classified as part of the variable costs of a prevention program. Expert opinion may be helpful in constructing a list of the resources that are needed to provide a particular service. The costs for materials and supplies can usually be obtained from the financial officer of the program. The cost of off-site laboratory tests can often be obtained from the state health department or the laboratory itself.

Materials and supplies cost per unit of service is determined by the following equation

$$\text{materials and supplies cost} = \text{specific resource} \times \text{cost per unit} \times \text{number of units used in time period} \tag{4}$$

Fixed Costs
Facilities and Space. Within a particular range of service volume, resources such as facilities, equipment, administrative support, and other direct costs are often paid in total and not per unit of service. For example, an X-ray machine may sit

idle some portion of every work day. If the X-ray machine was essential for screening, the same equipment cost would occur whether 10 or 20 participants were screened per day. (The cost of the film and supplies, of course, is a per-service expense.) Thus, the following calculations are suggested.

To determine the cost of *facilities*, the cost of facilities required to implement the program should include the cost of space, including maintenance costs, and the cost of utilities. If a program is to be conducted in an existing facility, the cost of the additional space and time needed for the new intervention is based on the proportion of the total time the facility is in use. The proportion of time and space needed for the new intervention should be multiplied by the total cost of space (e.g., rent, ownership, taxes, insurance, maintenance) plus the cost of utilities. If neither additional facilities nor additional time is used, i.e., a marginal analysis is being conducted, then the facility cost can be ignored.

Costs for facilities are usually recorded as either the cost per unit, e.g., cost per square foot, or the total cost for the facility, e.g., utility costs or insurance costs. When calculating costs within a portion of an existing facility, it is often useful to obtain the total square footage for the facility and convert all facility costs to the cost per square foot.

The following equations can be used to determine the facility's costs for programs sharing space in an existing facility.

$$\textit{facilities costs} = \textit{additional facility space used by the} \\ \textit{program} \times \textit{cost per square foot for space and utilities,} \qquad (5)$$

or

$$\textit{facilities costs} = (\textit{total facility cost for space and} \\ \textit{utilities} \div \textit{total facility time used, including program)} \\ \times \textit{facility time used by program} \qquad (6)$$

An example of each type of facility's cost calculation follows.

Example 1: A new workplace health education program uses 168 square feet of office space in a factory complex. The facility's cost for the complex is estimated at $30 per square foot per year including utilities. Using equation (5), the facility's cost for the worksite health education program is $5,040 (168 square feet × $30 per square foot).

Example 2: A worksite health education office decides to add a cholesterol screening program. The total facility's cost for the 168-square-foot health education office is $5,040 per year ($30 per square foot). The office is open 8 hours each day. The cholesterol screening program will be available for 1 hour each day. It will be the only service offered during that hour. Using equation (6), the facility's cost for the cholesterol screening program is $630 per year ($5,040 ÷ 8 hours per day) × (1 hour per day).

Capital Equipment and Real Estate. The implementation of prevention programs often involves the purchase of new or use of existing *capital equipment* and *real estate*. These costs are likely to occur only once during the lifetime of a program. Computing the costs of equipment and real estate associated with the intervention involves two steps:

1. Computing the equivalent annual cost
2. Computing the proportion of the equivalent annual cost that is assigned to the intervention

Two methods are recommended for computing the equivalent annual cost. The first and the simplest is to determine whether market rates exist for renting comparable buildings or for leasing comparable equipment. These rates can be used to estimate the annual cost of capital equipment or real estate. The second and more accurate method is to annuitize the initial outlay over the useful life of the asset. The method for annuitizing capital costs is presented in chapter 6. Another frequently used method for computing equivalent annual costs was developed by Richardson and Gafni.[8,10]

Administrative and Staff Support. Costs for administrative and staff support are calculated as a proportion of the staff time spent on this particular intervention. Salary and fringe benefits for each person who provides administrative and staff support are multiplied by the proportion of the person's time spent providing services for the intervention being studied.

The following equation is used to determine the cost of administrative and staff support associated with a program.

$$administration \ and \ support \ costs \ = \ [proportion \\ of \ administrators' \ time \ spent \ on \ intervention \ \times \\ (salary \ + \ benefits)] \ + \ [proportion \ of \ support \\ staff \ time \ spent \ on \ intervention \ \times \ (salary \ + \ benefits)] \qquad (7)$$

Volunteer Time. The major nonmarket resource (a resource not traded in a market and which therefore does not have a market price) in prevention programs is time spent by volunteers. Two approaches to accounting for volunteer time are frequently described in the health-care literature. The first approach assumes that a volunteer values his or her time spent in volunteer work as he or she would value leisure time. The most commonly used method for quantifying leisure time spent volunteering is to use one-half of the volunteer's wage rate. However, this method can have distinct distributional biases. Programs that rely on volunteers who are middle- or upper-income earners may appear very expensive.

To cope with this problem and to attempt to quantify volunteer time consistently, without regard for population characteristics, another method is recommended. With this method, the value of time spent in volunteer work is based on the equivalent wage rate of a person employed in a job that fits the description of the volunteer work.

Donated Goods and Services. In addition to volunteer time, programs frequently make use of other donated goods and services. These resources are also included in the cost inventory. The market value for these inputs is used as the cost of the resources. For example, resources for a bicycle helmet education program may include public service announcements for which both media production and airtime are donated. To estimate the cost of these resources, purchased production services and the cost of airtime can be used.

When reporting the results of intervention cost analyses in which a substantial portion of costs are allocated to volunteer time or other donated goods and services, these resources should be highlighted to indicate the extent to which a cost-effective intervention relies on nonfinancial inputs. Separate reporting of an intervention's financial and economic costs increases the generalizability of prevention-effectiveness studies by indicating the resources necessary to replicate an intervention regardless of whether the resource requires a financial outlay or is donated.

Participant Costs

The effectiveness of a prevention intervention may be influenced by out-of-pocket expenses incurred by a participant and a participant's time in receiving an intervention. Participant costs can be one of the largest costs associated with an intervention and should be included in intervention cost analyses conducted from the societal perspective. Costs for participants fall into two categories: out-of-pocket expenses and productivity losses. *Out-of-pocket expenses* are costs that participants incur for items such as travel and child care needed to allow participation in an intervention. Other out-of-pocket expenses include the purchase of items not accounted for in program costs such as purchase of bicycle helmets, dietary supplements, or condoms.

Productivity losses by participants are wages the participant does not receive because of time taken off from work to participate in the intervention. Productivity losses include costs assigned to travel time, waiting time, and actual service time for the participant.

One method for collecting participant costs is by participant survey. Survey data can be obtained by interviewing participants while they are present in a facility to receive an intervention. Information can be collected about travel, arrival time, and service time. Questions asked of the participants can include the following:

- How far did you travel (miles)?
- Where did you begin your travel (home, work, school . . .)?
- What time did you leave that place?
- What time did you arrive at the intervention site?
- What time did you leave the intervention site?
- What expenses did you incur in order to come to the intervention site, e.g., bus fare, tolls, mileage, child care?

The cost of participant time is based on average earnings. The analyst must decide whether to use average earnings figures for the U. S. population as an average, or earnings figures for the particular population of clients receiving the intervention. Participant productivity losses are calculated in the same manner as lost productivity from morbidity or premature mortality. Again, the analyst must decide whether to use participant-specific data or averages for the U. S. population. Appendix I lists average earnings in various categories for the U. S. population. Earnings data for participants may be obtained by surveys of actual program participants. Participant costs are calculated by multiplying the time for travel, waiting, and service by the average earnings. For explicit instructions on the use of the tables in Appendix I, see chapter 8.

To obtain total participant costs, participant productivity losses are added to out-of-pocket expenses (e.g., mileage or travel expenses, any child- or elder-care expenses, and any other cost paid by the participant). It may be desirable to present the out-of-pocket expenses and the participant productivity losses separately in the cost analysis. One exception to including participant produc-tivity losses in a prevention-effectiveness study is in a cost-utility analysis in which the utility measurement includes a quality adjustment for participation in an intervention. More on the subject of including productivity losses is pre-sented in chapters 7, 8, and 9.

The participant costs can be calculated using the following equation.

$$participation\ costs\ =\ (sum\ of\ the\ time\ that\ participants$$
$$spend\ traveling,\ waiting,\ and\ participating\ in\ the\ service$$
$$\times\ median\ salary)\ +\ (sum\ of\ the\ out\text{-}of\text{-}pocket\ expenses$$
$$participants\ accrue\ for\ participation) \tag{8}$$

Cost of Intervention Side Effects

Some interventions have adverse side effects as well as benefits. The benefits of an intervention must exceed the risks if the intervention is to meet an acceptable ethical standard. Costs associated with the side effects of an intervention must be included in any cost analysis and are counted as a cost of the intervention. For example, even an extremely small risk of a severe reaction following the administration of a vaccine must be included in the costs for a mass vaccination program, because with so many doses administered, there is a probability that an adverse side effect will occur. The costs associated with the probability of side effects need to be included.

The same methods for determining the cost of health outcomes averted are used to determine the costs of side effects. The method selected for measuring side effects will depend on the type of analysis—CBA, CEA, or CUA. Informa-tion on the probability of side effects and the resources required to treat persons who experience them can be found in the literature in epidemiologic studies and from experts. If the side effects substantially change or add to the relevant outcomes in the analysis, they should be incorporated into the structure of the decision tree. But, if the side effects are relatively minor and have an impact only on the cost of the intervention, such costs can be incorporated without modify-ing the structure of the decision tree. For example, gastrointestinal upset from single-dose antibiotic therapy to treat *Chlamydia trachomatis* may require an over-the-counter medication cost but does not have an impact on the on the effectiveness of the treatment and the subsequent health outcome—cases of pelvic imflammatory disease prevented. In this case, only the cost of the side effect may need to be included. However, if the treatment were a 10-day course of antibiotic therapy and the gastrointestinal upset led to discontinuation of the therapy, the effectiveness of the treatment may be diminished, decreasing the number of cases of PID prevented. In this case, because the side effects may have substantially changed the health outcome, the probability and impact of side effects should also be incorporated into the decision tree. It may also be desirable to structure the tree to allow the number of cases of side effects to be calculated. When conducting a CUA, if the side effects impinge upon an individual's quality of life, the model should be structured so that this impact is incorporated into the outcome measure, e.g., quality-adjusted life years gained.

CALCULATE TOTAL AND EXPECTED COST
OF THE INTERVENTION

Once each individual resource and its unit cost are calculated for the time period in question, including the annualization of capital inputs, the total and annual costs of the intervention can be calculated. To determine the average or marginal cost per intervention unit, the number of participants (or other output measures) served by each part of the intervention should be measured.

The calculation of total, annual, and average intervention cost involves the following steps:

1. Multiply the cost per unit by the number of units used for each resource in the time period to obtain the sum of the variable costs.
2. Sum the fixed costs for the time period.
3. Annualize and sum the capital costs for the time period.
4. Sum the subtotals from 1, 2, and 3; the participant costs for the time period; and any costs for side effects associated with intervention. This sum is the *total cost* of the intervention.
5. To convert the total cost of an intervention with a multiyear time period to a shorter time frame, divide the total cost by the number of years to obtain the *annual cost*. (Note that annual intervention costs that occur in years following the base year of the analysis should be discounted. See chapter 6.)
6. Divide the total cost by the number of participants or other relevant intervention unit to obtain the *average cost* of the intervention.
7. To calculate the *marginal cost* of the intervention, follow the steps above but exclude costs not relevant to the marginal analysis, i.e., fixed costs and capital costs.

Table 5.3 provides an example of a worksheet used to calculate total annual cost and average cost of an intervention. The worksheets provided at the end of the chapter will facilitate these calculations.

Table 5.3 A Worksheet for Calculating the Annual Cost and the Average Cost Per Client for a Hypothetical HIV Counseling Program

Resource	Quantity (A)	Cost/Unit (B)	Total Cost (A × B)
FIXED COSTS			
Personnel[a]			
Administrator	.05 years	64,421.00	3,221
Clerical worker	.13 years	14,375.00	1,869
Facilities			
Rent	12 months	1,485.00	17,820
Maintenance	12 months	240.00	2,880
Utilities	12 months	150.00	1,800
Phone	12 months	86.00	1,032
Supplies & Equipment			
Office supplies	12 months	450.00	5,400
Computer[b]	12 months	1,900.00	1,900
Subtotal			*35,922*
VARIABLE COSTS			
Personnel[a]			
Counselor (4 hours/session)	980 hours	22.44	21,991
Supplies & Misc.			
Client education materials	4,900 sets	2.80	13,720
Travel	11,000 miles	0.28	3,080
Participant Costs[c]			
Travel	58,800 miles	0.28	16,464
Subtotal			*55,255*
TOTAL			91,177
Participants per year (20 participants/session × 5 sessions/week × 49 weeks/year)			4,900
Total annual cost			91,177
Average cost per participant			18.61

[a] Includes benefits
[b] Annualized cost of capital equipment
[c] Productivity losses not included

CONCLUSION

This chapter has described the basic concepts, definitions, and techniques necessary to determine intervention costs in a prevention-effectiveness study. The issues associated with prospective, retrospective, and prevention-effectiveness models have been described. The process for establishing criteria for a cost inventory has been discussed. Costs have been categorized and collection techniques for program costs and participant costs have been described. Side effects of interventions have also been discussed. In chapter 6, the concepts and methods for adjusting costs that occur in different time periods are presented.

REFERENCES

1. Teutsch SM. A framework for assessing the effectiveness of disease and injury prevention. *MMWR* 1992;41 (No. RR-3):i–iv, 1–12.
2. Borus MEJ, Buntz CG, Tash WR. *Evaluating the impact of health programs: a primer.* Cambridge: The MIT Press, 1982.
3. Warner KE, Luce, BR. *Cost-benefit and cost-effectiveness analysis in health care.* Ann Arbor: Health Administration Press, 1982.
4. Drummond MF, Stoddart GL, Torrance GW. *Methods for the economic evaluation of health care programmes.* Oxford: Oxford University Press, 1987.
5. Luce BR, Elixhauser A. *Standards for socioeconomic evaluation of health care products and services.* New York: Springer-Verlag, 1990.
6. Petitti DB. *Meta analysis, decision analysis, and cost-effectiveness analysis: methods for quantitative synthesis in medicine.* New York: Oxford University Press, 1994.
7. Gorsky RD, Teutsch SM. Assessing the effectiveness of disease and injury prevention programs: costs and consequences. *MMWR* 1995;44 (No. RR-10):i–ii, 1–10.
8. Gorsky RD. A method to measure the costs of counseling for HIV prevention. *Public Health Rep* (in press).
9. Robinson R. Costs and cost-minimisation analysis. *Br Med J* 1993;307:726–28.
10. Richardson AW, Gafni A. Treatment of capital costs in evaluating health-care programs. *Costs and Management* Nov–Dec 1983: 26–30.

WORKSHEET FOR ESTIMATING PERSONNEL COSTS

Type of personnel	Number	Average annual salary or earnings (including benefits)	%time spent on program and project activities	Annual cost of personnel $
Salaried				
a)				
b)				
c)				
Subtotal				
Hourly				
a)				
b)				
c)				
Subtotal				
Volunteers*				
a)				
b)				
c)				
Subtotal				
TOTAL				

* The value of volunteer time can be estimated by determining the salaried or hourly wages required for a paid employee in that position.

DONATED RESOURCES & APPROACHES TO DETERMINING ECONOMIC COSTS

Donated Resources	Approach to determining economic costs	COSTS
a)		
b)		
c)		
d)		
e)		
f)		
g)		
h)		

WORKSHEET FOR CALCULATING SUPPLIES

Supplies	Amounts (A)	Costs (C)	TOTAL (A) x (C)
Subcategory 1*			
a)			
b)			
c)			
Subtotal			
Subcategory 2*			
a)			
b)			
c)			
Subtotal			
Subcategory 3*			
a)			
b)			
c)			
Subtotal			
TOTAL			

* Subcategories can include office, clinic, educational materials, etc.

WORKSHEET FOR RECORDING INTERVENTION COSTS
BY RESOURCE CATEGORY

Resource Category	(Annual) Economic Cost (Donated/In-kind)	(Annual) Financial Cost (Expenditures)	TOTAL
CAPITAL/START-UP			
Vehicles			
Equipment			
Buildings - Space			
Training - Non- Recurrent			
Other			
Subtotal			
RECURRENT/MAINTENANCE			
Personnel			
Supplies			
Vehicles - Oper. & Maint.			
Buildings - Oper. & Maint.			
Training - Recurrent			
Media			
Other Operating Inputs			
Subtotal			
TOTAL			

WORKSHEET FOR TRANSPORTATION COSTS

Capital/ Start-up	Purchase Price* (A)	Annualized Cost (B)	% of time used for program (C)	TOTAL (B) x (C)
Vehicle 1)				
Vehicle 2)				
Vehicle 3)				
Subtotal				

Recurrent/ Maintenance	Variable		Fixed	TOTAL
	unit (gal.,mile, etc.)	$/unit		
Lease				
Operation				
Maintenance				
Insurance				
Other				
Subtotal				
TOTAL ANNUAL TRANSPORTATION COSTS				

WORKSHEET FOR CALCULATING TOTAL PROGRAM COSTS

PROJECT YEAR:_____   LENGTH OF PROJECT (# of years): _____

Item	Unit of Analysis	# of Units	COSTS		
			Capital/ Start-up	Recurrent/ Fixed	Recurrent/ Variable

6

Time Preference

PHAEDRA A. SHAFFER
ANNE C. HADDIX

Invariably, the study of a prevention-effectiveness strategy will have costs and benefits spread out over multiple years. Economic costs and benefits from published data are often available from different years than the study. To determine the economic viability of an intervention, past and future costs and benefits must be adjusted and translated to their *present* value. In this chapter, we introduce the concept of differential timing of costs and benefits and the mechanics of discounting, inflation, and annuitization.

DEFINITION OF DISCOUNTING

Even in a world of zero inflation, there are advantages to incurring costs later or receiving benefits earlier. Thus it is necessary to incorporate the concept of *time preference* into a prevention-effectiveness analysis. The process of converting future costs and benefits into their present value is called *discounting*. The quantitative measure of time preference is the *discount rate*.

The cost of an intervention often is incurred in the present, but associated benefits (or the cost of illness averted) accrue only in the future. For example, if Program A has a cost of $100 in the first year and produces a benefit of $110 in the second year and Program B has a cost of $100 in the first year but yields a benefit of $105 in the first year, at first glance it may appear that Program A's net benefit outweighs Program B's net benefit by $5. However, society places a premium or a preference (reflected in the *discount rate*) on benefits received today versus benefits received in the future. To incorporate this preference, the present value (PV) of future costs or benefits is calculated by the process of discounting. In the example above, if a 10% discount rate is used, $110 in benefits in the second year would be discounted to a present value of $100 in the first year. When time preference is incorporated into the analysis, Program B's net benefits exceed Program A's by $5.

Many different discount rates have been used. Conceptually, the appropriate discount rate depends on the perspective of the study and the question posed by the study. Rates may be based on such factors as the market interest rates, the marginal productivity of investment, the corporate discount rate, the government rate of borrowing, the individual personal discount rate, or the social discount rate.

The discount rate for prevention-effectiveness studies that take the societal perspective is called a social discount rate. This is the rate at which society as a whole is willing to exchange present costs for future benefits. The social discount rate is based on the assumption that individuals in society get satisfaction from knowing that future society will "inherit" good health because of current investment in prevention, even though spending money in the present requires consumption trade-offs. Because of individuals' attitudes toward society, consideration of children as part of future society, and feelings of altruism toward humanity, the social discount rate is lower than an individual's personal discount rate or a private-sector discount rate. A low discount rate indicates that future benefits are also valued highly in the present. Because a social discount rate reflects the values of society as a whole, it is the most appropriate rate for public policy decisions. Krahn and Gafni provide a more thorough discussion of the types of discount rates and their application to economic evaluations of health care programs.[1]

If a prevention-effectiveness study takes a perspective other than a societal perspective, however, a discount rate other than the social discount rate might be selected. For example, if a study of a prevention intervention is undertaken from the perspective of a health maintenance organization (HMO), a private-sector discount rate might be used. The selection of such a rate reflects the assumption that HMOs make investment decisions based in part on the profitability of the intervention. An HMO may have a higher discount rate, indicating that averting costs in the present is preferred to averting costs in the future.

Once the appropriate type of discount rate is selected, the value of the rate must be chosen. There has been wide variation in the choice of a discount rate for studies taking the societal or the federal government perspective. The Office of Management and Budget issued guidelines in 1993 requiring that an 8% discount rate be used for assessing the costs and benefits of federal projects.[2] Studies of health-care interventions, also conducted from the societal perspective, have typically used a lower discount rate on the general premise that societal preferences for health improvements differ from consumer goods.[1] In his guide to cost-benefit analysis, Gramlich recommends a 4% discount rate.[3] Drummond et al. advocate a 5% rate as does Louise Russell in her 1986 book on prevention strategies.[4,5] A review of the Medline data base from 1988 to 1991 showed that the most common base-case rate in the health-care literature was 5%.[1] Recently, the Panel on Cost-Effectiveness in Health and Medicine, under the auspices of the Public Health Service, recommended that cost-effectiveness analyses of health interventions use a 3% discount rate.

To increase the comparability of the public health programs, this book recommends the use of either a 3% or a 5% *real* discount rate for both costs and benefits—monetary and nonmonetary. The term "real" indicates that this discount rate is free from the effects of inflation. When a real discount rate is used, all monetary costs and benefits are reported in *real* or *constant* dollars for a specific base year. Costs and benefits that will be incurred in the future are not adjusted for anticipated inflation. (See "Adjusting for Inflation" below.) Because the selection of the discount rate can influence the decision result, this text supports Weinstein and Stason's recommendation for wide sensitivity analysis on the discount rate.[6]

Recommendation: For the purposes of conducting economic analyses, it is recommended that either a 3% or a 5% real discount rate be used. No adjustments for inflation in the future should be made, because this is a *real* discount rate. Perform sensitivity analysis on the discount rate from 0% to 8%.

Discounting Dollars to Base-Year Monetary Units

The concept of discounting is similar to the concept of compounding interest. A compound interest rate is used to calculate the future value (FV) of money, i.e., how much will a sum of money invested today be worth in the future. The discount rate is the reverse of this and is used to calculate the present value (PV) of a sum of money to be received in the future. In the above example, the PV of $110 received 1 year from now is equal to $100 now, when the discount rate is 10%.

To calculate the PV of a future value, the *discount factor* is $(1 + r)^{-t}$, or

$$\frac{1}{(1 + r)^t} \tag{1}$$

and can be obtained for a given year (t) and discount rate (r) from Appendix G. Once the discount factor is known, this number can be multiplied by the future dollar amount to obtain the present dollar amount.

The equation for discounting a stream of future dollars into present value dollars is as follows:

$$PV = \sum_{t=0}^{N} F_1 (1 + r)^{-t} \tag{2}$$

or

$$PV = F_0 + \frac{F_1}{(1 + r)} + \frac{F_2}{(1 + r)^2} + \frac{F_3}{(1 + r)^3} + \ldots + \frac{F_n}{(1 + r)^n} \tag{3}$$

where

PV = present value
F = future value at year n
r = discount rate
t = time period
n = analytic horizon

If the stream of costs or benefits remains constant over time, i.e., the annual cost or the annual benefit is unchanged for a period of years, equation (4) can be used to calculate the present value of that stream. This equation is used in place of the year-by-year process as shown in (2) and (3).

$$PV = F \left[\frac{1}{r} - \frac{1}{r(1+r)^n} \right] \tag{4}$$

where

PV = present value
F = future annual value
r = discount rate
n = years of constant stream

Discounting Nonmonetary Benefits

As explained in the previous section, future monetary values are adjusted to present monetary values because of the time preference for money, i.e., a dollar now is worth more than a dollar in the future. Future health outcomes are also discounted, not because health outcomes realized today are more valuable than health outcomes realized tomorrow, but because in prevention-effectiveness studies, if health outcomes are not discounted but the costs are discounted, the cost per health outcome prevented will decrease over time. Thus discounting health outcomes at the same rate as monetary outcomes creates an "exchange rate" for dollars and health outcomes that is time invariant. For this reason, when nonmonetary health outcomes are discounted, they should be discounted at the same rate as dollars.[1,6,7] An undiscounted value can be used in the presentation of the study results when the health outcomes prevented are reported independently of the summary measure.

In addition to issues of logical consistency, a growing body of literature captures the continuing debate on the treatment of future health outcomes; the appropriate discount rate for health outcomes; individual preferences for health improvements compared to consumption goods; societal preference for health now versus later; and discounting intergenerational costs and benefits.[7-16] Many issues remain unresolved; research and discussion continue on this subject.

Weinstein and Stason present an example of the inconsistencies that arise when monetary costs are discounted and nonmonetary health outcomes are not discounted.[17] Assume that an investment of $100 today would result in saving 10 lives (or 1 life per $10 of investment). If the $100 were invested at a 10% rate of return, then 1 year from now the $100 would be worth $110. With $110, it would be possible to save 11 lives. In two years, the $100 original investment would net $121, and it would be possible to save 12 lives. On the basis of these calculations, the returns in the future look so appealing that one might never choose to save any lives in the present! To correct for this possible inconsistency, both monetary and nonmonetary benefits should be discounted at the same rate.

To attach greater value to the delayed benefits of prevention programs, some prevention-effectiveness practitioners argue that health outcomes should be discounted at a slightly lower rate than that used for costs. When this is done, prevention programs can be made to appear to be more cost-effective. However, there is no theoretical basis for this approach. The mechanism for discounting costs and benefits should be used to reflect the society's time preference, not to adjust the intrinsic value of health outcomes. Rather, if society indeed values the benefits of prevention programs, values assigned to health outcomes that will occur in the future discounted at the same rate as costs should reflect this preference.

Recommendation: Discount future nonmonetary health outcomes at 3% or 5% (the same rate as monetary costs and benefits). Perform sensitivity analysis from 0% to 10%.

ADJUSTING FOR INFLATION

When an economic analysis is done, data on cost are often collected from years besides the base year of the evaluation. To ensure that all costs are comparable and that costs can be weighed against benefits that occur in the same time period, it is necessary to standardize the costs to one time unit. Cost data reported for previous years can be adjusted for a specified base year by using either the Consumer Price Index (CPI) or a relevant subindex. The CPI is an explicit price index that directly measures movements in the weighted average of prices of goods and services in a fixed "market basket" of goods and services purchased by households over time. Appendix H presents the Consumer Price Index for all items and for the medical-care component for the period 1960–1994.

To adjust the cost of an item reported for a year before the base year, divide the index value for the base year by the index value for the year in which the cost was reported. Then multiply the result by the unadjusted value of the item. The formula for this calculation is

$$Y_B = Y_P \left[\frac{D_B}{D_P} \right] \tag{5}$$

where

Y_B = base year value
Y_P = past year value
D_B = index value of base year
D_P = index value of past year

For example, if data are available for the 1990 cost of a visit to a clinician but are needed for a study using 1992 costs, the cost of the visit to the clinician can be inflated to 1992 dollars, using the physician-services component of the CPI. The ratio of the 1992 to 1990 index values ($181.2/160.8 = 1.127$) is multiplied

by the cost of a 1990 visit to a clinician ($45), and the result is the cost of a visit
to a clinician in 1992 dollars ($51).

$$51 = 45 \left[\frac{181.2}{160.8} \right]$$

Adjusting Earnings to the Base-Year Monetary Units

Just as costs must be adjusted to base-year monetary units, earnings reported for
past years must also be adjusted to base-year monetary units. However, because
earnings do not increase and decrease at the same rates as prices, the CPI
should not be used. Instead, the adjustment of past years' earnings to base-year
monetary units uses the estimated annual increase in average hourly earnings
reported annually in the March issues of *Employment and Earnings* from the
U. S. Department of Commerce, Bureau of Labor Statistics. These data can
also be located in the most recent issue of the *Statistical Abstract of the United
States.*[18] The equation for adjusting earnings is

$$I_B = I_P \left[\frac{W_B}{W_P} \right] \tag{6}$$

where

I_B = income in base year
I_P = income in past year
W_B = average hourly wage in the base year
W_P = average hourly wage in the past year

For example, a cost-effectiveness analysis which includes productivity losses has
a 1993 base year. The productivity losses data are reported based on 1990
income. The average hourly earnings for 1990 and 1993 were $10.01 and
$10.83, respectively. Thus income of $23,582 in 1990 would be adjusted to
$25,514 for a 1993 base year by this calculation:

$$\$25,514 = \$23,582 \left[\frac{10.83}{10.01} \right]$$

ANNUITIZING CAPITAL EXPENDITURES

Several types of costs must be considered in evaluating prevention programs:
direct program costs, direct medical costs, and indirect costs. Direct program
costs can include the cost of personnel and materials categorized as ongoing
costs or start-up costs. Ongoing costs are the annual expenditures necessary to
keep a program running (e.g., payroll costs). Start-up costs are the one-time
capital expenditures necessary for the early implementation stage of a program.
These costs may include capital equipment costs. Although the costs of capital
expenditures occur at one time, the benefits accrue over their useful life. Since

capital investments such as for equipment are used over the duration of a project, the costs of capital expenditures may be spread out over that time period. This is done by annuitizing, i.e., determining an annual value of the capital item for the life of the capital investment. The annual value can then be used with other annual costs to calculate costs for the duration of a project.

Richardson and Gafni use two criteria for calculating the equivalent annual cost of a one-time capital expenditure.[19] The annuitizing of costs should be consistent with the present-value method of calculation used in the analysis. If 5% is used in the calculation of the discount factor to estimate the present value of future costs, then 5% should be used in the calculation of the annuity factor to estimate the equivalent annual cost of a one-time capital expenditure. Second, in annuitizing costs, the equivalent annual cost should yield a constant cost value for each year of the useful life of the capital. The equivalent annual cost can then be used to calculate costs for the duration of the project.

The method described below meets both criteria. First, the scrap value should be subtracted from the original purchase cost; the result should then be divided by the appropriate annuity factor. *Scrap value* refers to the resale value of the capital expenditure at the end of the project. Use of this method, which is simple and direct, avoids understatement or overstatement of annual costs, which could lead to incorrect decisions about the allocation of resources in health care. The equations for annuitizing a one-time capital expenditure are as follows:

$$C = \left[P - S\frac{1}{(1 + r)^t} \right] [A(t, r)]^{-1} \tag{7}$$

$$A(t, r) = \left[1 - \frac{1}{(1 + r)^t} \right] r^{-1} \tag{8}$$

where

C = calculated equivalent annual cost of the unit
P = cost of purchasing the unit
S = present value of the scrap value(after n years of service) of the unit
r = discount rate
$A(t,r)$ = annuity factor

Notice that in (8), in calculating the annuity factor,

$$\frac{1}{(1 + r)^t}$$

represents the discount factor. Once the appropriate discount rate (r) is determined and the useful life of the unit (t) has been determined, the discount factor can easily be determined by using the equation above. Appendix G provides discount factors from 1% to 10%. For comparability, either a 3% or a 5% discount rate should be used.

Once the discount factor is calculated, the annuity factor, $[A(t,r)]$, can be calculated by subtracting the discount factor from 1 and dividing by the discount rate, as shown in (8). An annuity table, listing annuity factors for n years of service and for discount rates from 1% to 10%, is provided in Appendix G.

The following example demonstrates the use of these formulas. The purchase price (P) of a new 6-test-tube centrifuge is $950. Assume the centrifuge will be used over 5 years and that its scrap value (S) after 5 years will be 20% of its original cost, or $190. The discount rate is 5%. Thus the present value of $190 in five years is $190 ÷ 1.05^5 or $149.

The next step is to calculate the appropriate annuity factor, using (8)

$$A(5, 0.05) = \left(1 - \frac{1}{(1 + 0.05)^5} \right) \ 0.05^{-1} = 4.33$$

Then the annual cost is calculated using (7):

$$\left((950 - 149) \ \frac{1}{(1 + 0.05)^5} \right) \ 4.33^{-1} = 144.94$$

When these methods are used to annuitize a one-time capital expenditure, a centrifuge purchased for $950 with a scrap value of $190 after 5 years has an equivalent annual cost of $144.94 over its 5-year life span.

CONCLUSION

This chapter has presented the three methods for adjusting costs and benefits, whether measured in monetary or nonmonetary terms, to the base year of the analysis. Discounting, adjusting for inflation, and annuitizing are methods used to adjust the costs of the intervention, the cost of the illness, and the costs of benefits.

REFERENCES

1. Krahn M, Gafni A. Discounting in the economic evaluation of health care interventions. *Med Care* 1993;5:403–18.
2. Office of Management and Budget. Circular no. A-94. *Guidelines and discount rates for benefit-cost analysis of federal programs.* 1992.
3. Gramlich EM. *A guide to benefit-cost analysis,* 2nd ed. Englewood Cliffs, NJ: Prentice-Hall, 1990.
4. Drummond MF, Stoddart GL, Torrance, GW. *Methods for the economic evaluation of health care programmes.* Oxford: Oxford University Press, 1987.
5. Russell LB. *Is prevention better than cure?* Washington, D.C.: The Brookings Institution, 1986.
6. Weinstein MC, Stasson WB. Foundations of cost-effectiveness analysis for health and medical practices. *N Engl J Med* 1977;296:716–21.

7. Keeler EB, Cretin S. Discounting of life-saving and other non-monetary effects. *Management Science* 1983;6:194–98.
8. Gafni A, Torrance GW. Risk attitude and time preference in health. *Management Sci* 1984;30:440–51.
9. Lipscomb J. Time preferences for health in cost-effectiveness analysis. *Med Care* 1989;27:Supp233–53.
10. MacKeigan LD, Larson LN, Draugalis JR, Bootman JL, Burns LR. Time preferences for health gains and health losses. *PharmacoEconomics* 1993;3:374–86.
11. Olsen JA. Time preferences for health gains: an empirical investigation. *Health Economics* 1993;2:257–66.
12. Redelmeier D, Heller D. Time preference in medical decision making and cost-effectiveness analysis. *Med Decision Making* 1993;13:212–17.
13. Weinstein M. Time-preference in the health care context. *Med Decision Making* 1993;13:218–19.
14. Ganiats TG. Discounting in cost-effectivness research. *Med Decision Making* 1994;14:298–300.
15. Redelmeier DA, Heller DN, Weinstein MC. Time preference in medical economics: science or religion? *Med Decision Making* 1994;14:301–3.
16. Torgerson DJ, Donaldson C, Reid DM. Private versus social opportunity cost of time: valuing time in the demand for health care. *Health Economics* 1994;3:149–56.
17. Weinstein MC, Stason WB. *Hypertension: a policy perspective.* Cambridge: Harvard University Press, 1976.
18. U. S. Bureau of the Census. *Statistical Abstract of the United States: 1994* (114th ed.) Washington, D.C., 1994.
19. Richardson AW, Gafni A. Treatment of capital costs in evaluating health-care programs. *Cost and Management* 1983;Nov–Dec:26–30.

BIBLIOGRAPHY

Alchian A. *Economic forces at work.* Indianapolis: Liberty Press, 1977.
Hartman, RW. One thousand points of light seeking a number: a case study of CBO search for a discount rate policy. *J Environmental Economics and Management* 1990;18(2):S3–S7.
Hellinger F. Forecasting the medical care costs of the HIV epidemic: 1991–1994. *Inquiry* 1991;28(Fall): 213–25.
Hodgson TA. State of the art of cost-of-illness estimates. *Adv Health Economics and Health Services Res* 1983;4:129–64.
Laidler D. *Introduction to microeconomics.* Oxford: Philip Allan Press, 1981.
Luce BR, Elixhauser A. Estimating costs in the economic evaluation of medical technologies. *Int J Technology Assessment in Health Care* 1990;6:57–75.
Lyon RM. Federal discount rate policy, the shadow price of capital, and challenges for reforms. *J Environmental Economics and Management* 1990;18:S29–50.
Phillips M. Why do costing? *Health Policy and Planning* 1987;2(3):255–57.
Scheraga JD. Perspectives on government discounting policies. *J Environmental Economics and Management* 1990;18:S65–71.
Tolpin HG, Bentkover JD. Economic costs of illness: decision-making applications and practical considerations. *Adv in Health Economics and Health Services Res* 1983;4:165–98.

7

Cost-Benefit Analysis

BETH CLEMMER
ANNE C. HADDIX

Cost-benefit analysis (CBA) is considered the "gold standard" of economic evaluation. It provides the most comprehensive consideration of the costs and benefits of intervention programs. The results of CBA are expressed in terms of net dollars. Because the common metric of dollars is used, CBA also provides a way to compare widely disparate programs in such areas as health, education, and the development of small businesses.

This chapter is one of three on economic analysis methods. It lays the foundation for subsequent chapters on cost-effectiveness analysis and cost-utility analysis.

COST-BENEFIT ANALYSIS DEFINED

CBA is a technique that attempts to value the consequences or benefits of an intervention program in monetary terms. Unlike CEA and CUA, which analyze outcome measures in terms of cost-per-unit-of-health-outcome, CBA attempts to place *dollar* values on program outcomes. All health outcomes are evaluated in CBA, whereas just one health outcome at a time is used in CEA.

In its simplest form, CBA attempts to weigh all the impacts of a program to assess whether it is worthwhile, i.e., whether its benefits exceed its costs. The results of CBA are reported as either the net present value (NPV), or net benefits of a project, or as the benefit-cost ratio. The formula for the NPV is

$$NPV = \sum_{t=0}^{T} \frac{(Benefits - Costs)}{(1 + r)^t}$$

where

r = discount rate
t = time period
T = time frame

Traditionally, CBA takes a societal perspective. Unlike other types of economic analyses used to assess the effectiveness of prevention strategies, CBA includes *all* costs and *all* benefits of an intervention program to identify programs that produce the largest social good. Because CBA is rooted in welfare economics, decisions are determined on the basis of economic efficiency, i.e., whether there is an aggregate net cost or net savings. Although CBA, CEA, and CUA all allow comparison among various health-program options, CBA is the only method that allows comparison of a *health* program with a *nonhealth* program in terms of economic resources.

CBA is often useful when a proposed public health intervention produces both a health and a nonhealth outcome. For example, a community-based lead-abatement program to reduce blood-lead levels in children may also increase local property values. The value of the benefit of increased property values would also be included in the analysis.

BACKGROUND OF COST-BENEFIT ANALYSIS IN HEALTH

CBA was first proposed as a technique to assist public policy decision making in 1844 in the essay "On the Measurement of the Utility of Public Works," by Jules Dupuit.[1] In the United States, the application of CBA began when Congress passed the United States Flood Control Act of 1936, which declared that benefits "to whomsoever they may accrue" of federal projects should exceed the costs. The first guidelines for conducting CBAs were issued in 1952 by the Bureau of the Budget. CBA has been widely used as a policy tool by the federal government ever since, particularly in the funding of public works projects and environmental regulations.

Early efforts to quantify health benefits and the value of life in monetary terms date from the seventeenth century.[2] However, the application of CBA in the health arena did not begin in earnest until 1966, when Dorothy Rice published her work on methods to estimate the cost of illness.[3] During the 1970s and early 1980s, applications of CBA for medical decision making appeared frequently in the literature.[4–8] However, because of the controversy over the valuation of health benefits, particularly the value of life, cost-effectiveness analysis rapidly became the most widely used technique for health-care decision making. Recently, because of the inability of CEA to fully capture the benefits of improved health, interest in CBA has been renewed. Current efforts are concentrated on refining benefits valuation methodology.[9–12]

WHEN TO USE COST-BENEFIT ANALYSIS

An analytic method must be appropriate to each particular prevention-effectiveness study. CBA is used to (1) decide whether to implement specific programs, (2) choose among competing options, or (3) set priorities on options within resource constraints. Generally, the CBA method is used before a public health program is implemented to evaluate whether the program produces a net savings. However, CBA can also be used to evaluate what has been accomplished by existing programs. Because CBA converts all costs and benefits into the common metric of dollars, CBA is also useful when an intervention produces multiple health outcomes. Although the conceptual structure of CBA is not difficult to understand, the actual design and implementation of this analytic method can be quite complex. From a practical standpoint, CBA is most useful in assessing programs for which accepted methods exist to quantify benefits in monetary terms.

LIMITATIONS OF CBA

CBA is an analytic tool with its own set of limitations. Many health-care interventions such as therapy for cancer, AIDS research, and treatments for end-stage renal disease often do not lend themselves readily to CBA because of difficulties in assessing the quality of health outcomes or in assigning a monetary value to a human life. Some intervention programs, such as programs to protect civil rights or to implement legally mandated requirements, achieve results that cannot readily be expressed in terms of economic efficiency. For such programs, a positive NPV determined by CBA may be a necessary, but not a sufficient, criterion for implementing a program. However, evaluation of a program in an emotionally and politically sensitive area with methods such as CBA, CEA, and CUA can help to make the costs and outcomes explicit, thereby adding clarity to discussion.

When used appropriately, CBA can provide important information for decision making. However, CBA does not make decisions; and it does not eliminate the need for judgment in public health decision making. For example, in addition to economic costs, policymakers must also look at issues such as distributional impacts—the potentially disparate impact of various proposals. CBA is a tool to *aid* decision making. If the analysis is done correctly, CBA clarifies the process of decision making and allows decision makers to examine the underlying criteria for selecting options.

The usefulness of CBA depends largely on the presentation of uncertainties in the analysis. Analyses that directly address uncertainties and report a range of estimates in sensitivity analyses are most useful, because they provide comprehensive information for further analysis and interpretation by decision makers.

Because CBA uses the common metric of dollars to express program outcomes, CBA answers one question that CEA and CUA cannot, i.e., "does a project generate net savings?" CEA and CUA generally compare options to find the least costly method of achieving a similar health outcome. CBA, however, also allows comparison of alternate strategies that have different outcomes. This is because in CBA all impacts are expressed in terms of dollars. Thus CBA can be used to compare alternate strategies that have very different outcomes, such as those related to health, education, or trade.

CBA evaluates the impact of a proposed project over the complete project period; however, it does not necessarily evaluate the internal efficiency of a project. CBA cannot determine whether the proposed method or another method would maximize social benefits. CBA simply determines whether the NPV is greater than zero or whether the benefit-cost ratio is greater than 1, i.e., whether the benefits exceed the costs. CBA provides a mechanism to compare different options to determine which projects have the highest NPV or benefit-cost ratio.

MANAGING LIMITATIONS OF CBA

CBA, like every other valuation method, has inherent weaknesses that have caused considerable controversy. As with any method of analysis, faulty assumptions or faulty estimates of impact invalidate the economic models created. In CBA, a set of external conditions in which the project will be conducted is assumed. If these assumptions are incorrect or if they change, the quality of the analysis is jeopardized. For example, unforeseen advances in medical technology could have an impact on some program options so that a model no longer accurately reflects the current range of possible options.

As with all economic models, the results of CBA are only as useful and precise as the information used in the calculations. The best ways to address uncertainty in the structure of the analysis and in the values of the model variables are by (1) subjecting the model and its assumptions to peer review, and (2) conducting sensitivity analyses (see below).

Perhaps the greatest problem in CBA is the assignment of a monetary value to human life or to a change in the quality of life that results from an illness or injury. In health, this issue is particularly sensitive, since public health programs often have a mandate to reduce unnecessary morbidity and premature mortality. If CBA is used, the savings in unnecessary morbidity and premature mortality are converted to a dollar value. From an ethical and moral perspective, human life is often considered priceless, so attempting to "value" it is difficult.

To avoid this controversy, investigators often use CEA rather than CBA. CEA forces policymakers to impute subjectively the value of a life without specifying a dollar value. However, it is important to remember that just because explicit dollar values are not assigned to lives in a CEA, determining a value for cost per life saved requires the user of the study, rather than the analyst, to place some value on those lives. Thus an advantage to CBA is that it makes certain assumptions explicit that remain implicit in other types of economic analysis.

Another apparent difficulty with CBA is that the techniques appear precise and objective. If users are not familiar with the underlying assumptions, the results can easily be misinterpreted and misused. The results are only as good as the analysis, assumptions, and valuations used and must be skillfully interpreted when used for decision making.

BASIC STEPS FOR A CBA

Following the guidelines in the previous chapters, there are nine basic steps to conducting a CBA:

- Frame the problem
- Identify the program or programs to be analyzed
- List the effects of the program for the full range of health and nonhealth outcomes in terms of benefits and costs
- Assign values (usually dollars) to the intervention and the outcomes
- Construct the decision tree
- Identify the probabilities
- Calculate the NPV of the program
- Evaluate results with sensitivity analyses
- Prepare the results for presentation

Frame the Problem

The first step in any economic analysis is to frame the question to be considered. Several decisions need to be made. The study question must be clearly stated. The perspective, time frame, and analytic horizon need to be specified. Each of these points was covered in chapter 2.

Identify the Project

The programmatic options to be considered are often specified by someone other than the analyst performing the CBA. As a first step, the analyst must decide on the scope of the analysis. Some questions to ask include:

- What is the general problem identified?
- What specific questions need to be answered?
- What are the options? (Even if there is no explicitly stated option, the analysis would compare the proposed project with the status quo. If there are various ways of accomplishing the same goal, first select options that are believed to be potentially cost-effective. Then vary the options as widely as possible to obtain the broadest comparison.)
- What differences among the options may affect comparability?
- Is CBA a reasonable methodology to use?

This last point is not always addressed. Questions to consider include:

- How large a project is being evaluated?
- How many uncertainties exist in terms of impact?
- Will it be acceptable to quantify all outcomes in monetary terms?

As stated earlier, CBA generally works well in a framework that is narrow enough to allow reasonable estimation of the major impacts of the project being evaluated.

Program Outcomes

Generally, since CBA takes a societal perspective, it is important to identify potential effects on all affected parties. At this stage, it is important to look beyond the outcomes that have readily available data and to include the entire set of program outcomes.

Identifying Outcomes
The identification of program outcomes is not as straightforward as it might seem. For example, if the primary health outcome is "morbidity prevented," then "life years saved" should not be the primary outcome measure of interest. If alleviation of pain and suffering has not been considered, treatment for such chronic disabling conditions as arthritis may never appear to be a desirable option. When evaluating diagnostic technologies, the analyst must often report intermediate outcome measures such as numbers of cases identified, since the effect on the incidence and prevalence of the condition and on the pattern of severity for these cases cannot be readily estimated. It may be impossible to substantiate the link between the intervention and the final outcome, because of lack of data, a long time lag between the intervention and the health outcomes, or confounding influences.

Common health-related benefits to be considered are

- Increased life expectancy
- Decreased morbidity
- Reduced disability
- Improved quality of life
- Averted medical costs
- Increased worker productivity

Nonhealth Outcomes
Often, public health programs yield benefits other than improved health. Such benefits might include improvement of environmental quality or increases in property values. The value of these benefits should also be included. When nonhealth benefits are not fully captured in the analysis, the net present value of the project will not reflect the total economic value gained by society if the proposed public health intervention is undertaken. CBA is often a useful method when it is desirable to include nonhealth benefits, because it allows different types of benefits to be measured with a common metric. Analysts must be careful not to attempt to achieve a positive net present value based on the inclusion of health benefits alone.

Intangible Outcomes
Some intangible outcomes, e.g., pain and suffering, may be critical to the analysis, and even though a perfect estimate cannot be obtained, such outcomes must be included. Some analysts err by including only benefits and costs that have been addressed in previous studies. Although this may be a good starting point, a credible analysis must include *all* relevant outcomes.

The issue of intangible costs and benefits is a difficult analytical problem. Certain outcomes cannot be valued neatly, but they must be evaluated or at least discussed. The willingness-to-pay (WTP) approach is often used to capture this aspect of a health outcome. This method of valuing outcomes is discussed in more detail below.

In many cases, an outcome can be assessed in terms of benefits or costs. For example, a medical cost averted can reasonably be classified as a benefit or as a "negative cost." The way in which an impact is classified may influence the results of CBA. If the summary measure for the analysis is the net-present-value calculation rather than benefit-cost ratio, it is not as important whether an impact is classified as a benefit or a cost. For a discussion of classification of impacts, see the section on "Summary Measures" below.

Valuation of Costs and Benefits

After the outcomes of the program are determined, values or dollar amounts are assigned to the outcomes and the cost of the intervention. Prevention-effectiveness studies often include values for (1) the intervention program, (2) any side effects, (3) the illness or injury prevented, and (4) other nonhealth outcomes. For a complete discussion of determining the costs of the intervention, see chapter 5. Any benefits or costs that occur after the first year of a program must be adjusted by discounting, as discussed in chapter 6.

When listing different costs and outcomes, benefits and costs must not be counted more than once. For example, to calculate the cost of a participant's time in a study, it is tempting to value both the participant's time as lost wages and the fee paid to that person to participate in the study. However, using both measures would constitute double counting, i.e., would include two measures of the volunteer's time. Only one of the two measures should be used to classify this cost. Since the volunteer is willing to participate for the fee paid, this measure might be considered one estimate of the value of volunteer time. (The fee may, of course, also include other inducements to overcome discomfort of a procedure or risk associated with participation in the study.) If wage rates are selected as a measure, they also need to be adjusted, because full wage rates will probably overestimate the costs of volunteer participation, since most people do not expect to receive their full wages to compensate for leisure-time activities.

Valuation of Health Outcomes

Valuation of costs and benefits for which market prices do not exist presents many problems. Some estimation techniques to deal with this difficulty include:

- Expert opinion: a delphi or consensus process can be used to determine the "best estimate" of professionals in the field
- Past policy decisions: estimates from previous legislative decisions may imply a certain baseline value
- Court awards: although court awards provide an estimate of some intangibles such as pain and suffering, court awards are often inconsistent, and thus are seldom used
- Cost-of-illness approach: a method for determining the economic cost of disease by summing the medical and nonmedical costs of the disease

and the productivity losses from associated morbidity or premature mortality

- Willingness-to-pay (WTP) approach: a method for determining how much people are willing to pay to decrease their risk of death or injury

The disadvantage to the first three approaches is that it is difficult to validate estimates and to separate other effects that contribute to the estimates. The cost-of-illness approach, although it can be validated, excludes any value of life beyond an individual's production potential and therefore may create a downward bias in estimates of the value of benefits (see chapter 8). To overcome these problems, the WTP approach is most frequently used in CBA. This method is described in the next section. Table 7.1 lists the strengths and weaknesses of the two methods. A more complete comparison of alternative valuation methods is presented by Fisher, Chestnut, and Violette.[12]

Willingness-To-Pay

The willingness-to-pay method (WTP) attempts to measure the value an individual places on reducing the risk of death or illness by estimating the maximum amount an individual would pay in a given risk-reducing situation. This method has a great deal of theoretical appeal, since the interests of a broad range of individuals are considered, including those who are not directly involved in decisions associated with the proposed project.

Rather than the value of the health outcome to any particular individual, this method assesses the value of a statistical health outcome (i.e., a statistical life) by determining what society as a whole is willing to pay to reduce by a certain amount the risk for each individual. The following example is taken from Fisher, Chestnut, and Violette: "If each of 100,000 persons is willing to pay $20 for a reduction in risk from 3 deaths per 100,000 people to 1 death per 100,000 people, the total WTP is $2 million and the value per statistical life is $1 million (with 2 lives saved)."[12]

Because there is no market pricing mechanism for reducing the risk of health outcomes, methods have been developed to determine societal WTP. Generally, WTP studies fall into three categories: required compensation or wage-risk studies, consumer market studies, and contingent market studies. Contingent market studies are most frequently used in the health economics arena. A short description of each method follows.

Required Compensation. The required-compensation approach attempts to look at the difference in wages for persons in occupations associated with higher risks than in other occupations. For example, again from Fisher, Chestnut, and Violette: "Suppose jobs A and B are identical except that workers in job A have higher annual fatal injury risks such that, on average, there is one more job-related death per year for every 10,000 workers in job A than in job B, and workers in job A earn $500 more per year than those in job B. The implied value of a statistical life is then $5 million for workers in job B who are each willing to forgo $500 per year for a 1-in-10,000 lower annual risk."[12]

Table 7.1   Strengths and weaknesses of COI and WTP*

Strengths	Weaknesses
COI	
COI is simple, concrete, and understood; measures resources currently spent by society	There may not be a close association between society's WTP to avert illness and COI
Permits aggregation of the full distribution of illness and death outcomes	Depends on incidence and severity of conditions being evaluated
Based on market-observed costs of medical services and wages	Difficulty measuring productivity losses for non-wage earners, undervalued workers, lives lost
Facilitates comparison of costs across health outcomes	Lower bound, since omits cost of lost leisure, pain and suffering, self-protection actions
	Measures what individuals say, rather than what they do
WTP	
More consistent with consumer demand theory than COI	Limited studies; results not yet widely validated
Easy to examine a sub-sector of the population	Potential for sample and question bias; results in questionable generalizability
Allows comparison of consumer preferences	Aggregation problem; results of WTP on a population basis may be misleading
Permits gathering of consumer preferences for alternate risk-reduction strategies, such as increase in self-protection actions	

*Adapted from "The Cost-of-Illness Method and the Social Costs of *Escherichia coli* O157:H7 Food-borne Disease." Tanya Roberts and Suzanne Marks, Economic Research Service, USDA.

This approach, like every other, has some drawbacks. For example, workers may not be aware of an increased risk and thus may not be able to evaluate wage rates in that context. If alternatives to workers' current job do not exist, compensation levels may not reflect the true rate of risk. Intangible costs such as pain and suffering of family members or dependents may not be captured in this measure. Also, a selection bias may exist toward individuals who practice high-risk behavior. Required compensation is a good first approximation of WTP for reducing statistical risks to life.

Consumer-Market Studies. The value of nonmarket resources can be imputed from reference to similar commodities for which a market exists. This method is similar to required compensation and suffers from the same limitations. Although work is progressing on this method, the seriousness of the drawbacks currently precludes its usefulness in health studies.

Contingent-Valuation Studies. The most reliable and frequently used method for estimating the WTP values of health outcomes is contingent valuation. Values were derived from surveys of individuals conducted in the context of a hypothetical market situation. Estimates are derived of mean or median WTP for a particular intervention designed to reduce the risk of a specific health outcome. To determine the value of benefits of a project, the mean or median WTP estimate is multiplied by the size of the population that receives the intervention. Because factors such as age, income, and education may influence an individual's WTP for a particular intervention, regression analysis is used to account for these influences.

The primary disadvantage of the contingent-valuation technique is that estimates are derived on the basis of what people say rather than what they do. However, surveys of the WTP and the contingent-valuation literature reveal that it is possible to achieve consistent and similar estimates for the value of specific health conditions.

Finally, contingent-value estimates of WTP may tend to undervalue the medical-cost component of the cost to society of an illness, because individuals with health insurance may not bear the full cost of their illness. This may have a disproportionately greater relative impact on the WTP to avoid aggravation of angina, than for an ailment such as a headache or cough, since angina may be associated with higher treatment costs.

The final section in this chapter provides a simple example of a cost-benefit analysis using the contingent-market approach to measure benefits. This example attempts to demonstrate the use of the contingent market method to obtain the measure of net benefits of the proposed program. It is in no way representative of the complexity of a real contingent-market study.

In general, for CBA, it is suggested that the WTP approach be used *only* when adequate survey instruments can be developed and when the WTP method is judged to be the best method for capturing significant nonmarket benefits or when reliable and comparable estimates are not available in the literature. For example, nonmarket benefits would be captured in a CBA of a regulatory program to reduce food-borne illness, where the WTP may provide the best estimate of the value society places on a safe food supply.

Limitations of WTP. The WTP method presents some difficulties. For example, wealthy individuals may be willing to pay more than economically disadvantaged individuals, simply because wealthy people *can* pay more. Also, people who are sick may be willing to pay more than healthy people. Most of the estimation techniques that examine value of life also have the drawback of assigning more value to some lives than others.

Although there are problems with the WTP method, the unsatisfactory alternative to this method is not to consider these issues at all. Refinements in WTP methodology are continuing, and more consistent estimates on the value of lives saved should be achievable. In current studies, it is most important to identify underlying assumptions and to make them explicit within the analysis.

Valuation of Benefits

One of the advantages of cost-benefit analysis is the ability to incorporate multiple outcomes into the analysis. Thus, the method is capable of aggregating across health outcomes and is particularly suitable in the evaluation of public health programs that also provide quantifiable nonhealth benefits. It is important not to exclude these from the analysis. For example, the positive NPV of a recent cost-benefit analysis of providing municipal water to areas along the U.S.–Mexico border hinged on the inclusion of the change in property values as a result of the project. References in the bibliography at the end of the chapter describe additional methods for valuing nonhealth benefits.

How far should one go in the valuation of other outcomes? The answer to this question depends on the purpose of the study and the intended user of the study results. If a program shows net benefits when only obvious benefits are included, it may not be necessary to continue to seek estimates of all benefits. However, if the time and the cost of gathering information can be justified, an attempt should be made to estimate dollar values for the major outcomes. Depending on initial results, the value of compiling additional data needs to be determined.

Although limiting data collection and accepting a noninclusive list of benefits may be expedient, there is some danger in this practice. If some benefits of a program are not valued, the program evaluated may lose perceived importance because benefits will be reduced in subsequent net-benefits calculations. It is important that all nonquantified impacts be highlighted in the presentation of results and interpretation of findings. Some studies have simply presented non-quantified impacts along with monetary estimates quantified on their own scales, e.g., as years of disability saved. These nonmonetary estimates are then excluded from the calculation of NPV. When benefits are not included, this fact should be mentioned in the discussion or conclusion.

Common Mistakes in Assessing and Valuing Benefits

Several common mistakes are made in assessing impact or valuation of impacts, including:

- Using dollar valuations of costs or benefits blindly, e.g., using hospital charges to represent medical costs
- Failing to account for all benefits
- Making assumptions about the effectiveness of the program. (The same level of health benefits may not be achieved during the start-up stage as in ongoing operation)
- Including benefits or costs that are not linked to the program and that therefore would have occurred without the program
- Double counting of costs and benefits
- Extrapolating from a small, biased sample to the whole population

Constructing the Decision Tree and Identifying Probabilities

The next two steps are to construct the decision model and identify the probabilities. Construction of the decision tree may be the most critical step of the analysis. This is the process by which nodes are mapped out and values are assigned to them. This step was described in chapter 3. This section focuses on construction details and data requirements for using this analytic framework to conduct a CBA.

A cost-benefit analysis uses a combination of epidemiologic and economic data. The first step in data collection is usually a thorough review of the literature. In the ideal analysis, data would be available from randomized, controlled trials or other well-designed studies that have undergone peer review and have been published in the scientific literature. Practically speaking, there are often gaps in the data that must be filled. One way that a gap can be filled is by conducting a study to answer the relevant question. However, this is often impossible, owing to time and resource constraints, and is frequently unnecessary. These gaps may also be filled by using an expert panel to develop estimates, or values can be assigned on the basis of available evidence. If these methods are used, the variables must be viewed as being uncertain and should be subjected to sensitivity analysis. Those that are critical to the results of the CBA may require further study.

The tree itself can be constructed using decision-analysis or spread-sheet software. First, the measures of effectiveness and the risk variables are expressed as probabilities in the decision tree. Then, the net cost of the branch is assigned as the value of the terminal node. The net cost is the sum of the costs and benefits of all events that occur on the path from the decision node to the terminal node. The difference in the expected costs of alternative interventions is the incremental NPV of benefits.

Analyzing the Model and Interpreting the Results

Once the tree or the spread sheet has been constructed, the model can be analyzed. The decision software programs will perform the averaging-out-and-folding-back function described in chapter 3 to determine the expected cost of each program option per individual or cohort. These expected costs can then be used to calculate the NPVs and incremental NPVs.

Net-Present-Value Calculations

A program passes the efficiency test and is considered worthwhile if the NPV of the program is positive. In the following calculation, a project is considered efficient if the result is greater than zero:

> Program Efficiency:
> PV of total benefits − PV of total costs = NPV > 0

where PV = present value.

When choosing among options, the program with the greatest NPV is preferable.

It is still common within the health literature to see benefit-cost or cost-benefit ratios reported as summary measures. With this approach, program decisions are made by taking the benefits of the program and dividing them by the costs. If the resulting ratio is greater than 1, the benefits exceed the costs, and the program is acceptable. However, this measure can also provide misleading answers. An example is shown in Table 7.2. In this example, the benefit-cost (B:C) ratio of Program A appears to be preferable. However, Program A only provides an NPV of $9, whereas the NPV of Program B is approximately $8,000. If one can afford the $2,000 investment, greater benefits will accrue from Program B.

Another disadvantage of expressing results as benefit-cost ratios is that the B:C ratio is also very sensitive to whether an impact is termed a benefit or a cost. For example, medical costs averted can be called a "negative cost" or a "benefit." In an NPV calculation, it does not matter how these costs are classified. In a B:C ratio, however, the numerator and denominator will vary considerably depending on the classification used. Because a B:C ratio may give a misleading answer, it is recommended that the NPV be used as the summary measure for evaluating program options.

Recommendation: The net present value of benefits, rather than a benefit-cost ratio should be used as the summary measure in a cost-benefit analysis.

Incremental Summary Measures

Cost-benefit analyses most commonly report the NPV or the B:C ratio of the intervention evaluated against the "no program" alternative. The formula for the NPV is

$$\text{AVG NPV} = (\text{PV Benefit}_A - \text{PV Benefit}_0) - (\text{PV Cost}_A - \text{PV Cost}_0)$$
$$A = \text{Program A}$$
$$0 = \text{no program}$$

It may be useful to report incremental results when evaluating a set of options. An incremental NPV is the additional benefit of one program over another minus the additional cost of the first program over the second. An incremental benefit-cost ratio is the additional benefit of one program over another divided by the additional cost of the first program over the second. Either measure provides information on the impact of an additional investment into the strategy with the next most costly intervention. The formula for the incremental NPV is

$$\text{INC NPV} = (\text{PV Benefit}_B - \text{PV Benefit}_A) - (\text{PV Cost}_B - \text{PV Cost}_A)$$
$$A = \text{Program A}$$
$$B = \text{Program B (the next most effective program)}$$

Table 7.2 Comparison of Net-Present-Value and Benefit-Cost Ratios

	Program A	Program B
Costs	$ 1	$ 2,000
Benefits	$10	$10,000
NPV	$ 9	$ 8,000
Benefit/cost ratio	10	5

In analyses when only one strategy is compared with no intervention, the NPV and incremental NPV for the cost-benefit analysis is the same.

Recommendation: When a cost-benefit analysis is used to evaluate more that one intervention strategy, the incremental NPV should also be reported.

Sensitivity Analyses

Because cost-benefit analyses are based on estimates and assumptions, sensitivity analyses should be performed to determine which variables exert the greatest influence on the results of the analysis. The robustness of the results can be determined so that critical variables can be identified and evaluated. For example, the choice of a discount rate may greatly affect an NPV calculation. When benefits accrue in the distant future, using a low discount rate makes programs appear more beneficial than using a higher discount rate. A description of sensitivity analyses was provided in chapter 3.

Depending on the number of benefits in an analysis, extensive sensitivity analyses may also be necessary to test the impact of assumptions and methodologies used for valuing these benefits. For these reasons, it is recommended that multivariable sensitivity analyses be performed and reported on a CBA model.

Recommendation: Multivariable sensitivity analyses should be performed and the results reported for a cost-benefit analysis.

Sensitivity analysis can identify the costs and benefits that most likely change the interpretation of the NPV calculation of a CBA, i.e., from negative to positive or vice versa. For instance, if varying the value of a single benefit measure for which there is uncertainty changes the NPV calculation, less certainty may exist about the conclusion. In this case, results of the sensitivity analyses must be highlighted in the presentation of findings.

Conversely, sensitivity analysis can also demonstrate when an assumption does not substantially affect a study conclusion. In this case, the decision maker may have more confidence in the results of the model. In addition, areas in need of further research can be identified through sensitivity analyses by identifying variables that have the greatest effect on the analysis.

Variables to Test in Sensitivity Analyses

Common variables in health care that should be tested with sensitivity analyses are

- Patient acceptance of or compliance with a program
- Risk of the disease or injury
- Discount rate
- Direct costs of the intervention
- Other costs
- Value of benefits

Threshold analysis, best- and worst-case-scenario analysis, and Monte Carlo simulations are also useful techniques to evaluate uncertainty (see chapter 3).

Presentations of Results

Because many analysts will make recommendations based on CBA, it is important to prepare results in a straightforward and useful form for decision makers. The presentation should include the following:

- Clearly defined question answered by the analysis
- Description of the options considered in the analysis
- Concise listing of the relevant outcomes considered for each option
- Explanation of valuation of outcomes with particular attention to estimation of intangible costs and benefits and differences in timing (discounting)
- Discussion of the evaluation of results with sensitivity analysis. (This is particularly important because it gives decision makers a sense of the robustness of the analysis so they can determine what weight the findings should be given)

AN EXAMPLE OF A CBA USING WTP ESTIMATION

Suppose you want to conduct a cost-benefit analysis of the use of household water vessels to prevent diarrhea. You decide to use the WTP approach to measure the benefits of the program. You conduct a contingent-valuation survey in a village of 100 households. You explain the use of the vessel in such a way that the villagers are clear that they are being asked to value the trade-off in their resources between either using a water vessel or coping with diarrhea in their household. You find the following:

5	households are WTP	$25 =	$125	(5%)
10	households are WTP	20 =	200	(15%)
50	households are WTP	15 =	750	(65%)
15	households are WTP	10 =	150	(80%)
15	households are WTP	5 =	75	(95%)
5	households are WTP	0 =	0	(100%)

From this information, you calculate that the median willingness-to-pay is $15.

Suppose that the vessel costs $10. You want to achieve an 80% coverage rate with the program so you decide to make the vessel available for $10. The total cost of the program is $800 (80 households × $10). The total benefits of the program are $1,225 ($125 + $200 + $750 + $150). The NPV of the program is $425 ($1,225 − $800). The concept here is that if a household has to pay only $10 for benefits they value at $25 then they get a surplus of $15 from the purchase. In economics, this is called *consumer surplus*. It is what CBA attempts to measure.

Now, you wish to consider increasing coverage to 95% of village households. You decide to lower the price to $5. Since the vessel costs $10, you give a $5 per vessel subsidy to the manufacturer. The program now costs $950. The total benefit is $1,300. The NPV of the program is $350.

The marginal NPV tells a different story. The additional benefit from an increase in coverage from 80% to 95% is $75 (15 × $5). The additional cost is $150 (15 × $10). The marginal NPV is − $75; expanding the program from 80% coverage to 95% generates a net loss.

CONCLUSION

CBA is the most comprehensive method of economic analysis and attempts to weigh all of the outcomes associated with a program's to determine whether that program's benefits exceed its costs. Because the results of CBA are expressed as dollars, programs with a variety of health outcomes and programs with different areas of impact may more easily be compared when CBA is used than when CEA and CUA are used.

The greatest area of controversy for CBA, CEA, and CUA is how to value reductions in risks to statistical lives and how to value changes in the quality of life. CBA assigns a monetary value to reducing risks to human life by several methods presented in this chapter. Assigning monetary values to changes in the quality of life is even more difficult; instead, it is usually omitted from CBA and listed as an intangible. However, as the methodology for CBA continues to develop, this method may be used more frequently for prevention-effectiveness studies.

CHECKLIST FOR COST-BENEFIT ANALYSIS

1. Has the program been clearly identified?
2. Have the specific questions to be answered been identified?
3. Have all reasonable options been clearly stated?
4. Is CBA the appropriate methodology for the study?
5. Have all outcomes of the program been identified?
6. Have the assumptions been specified?
7. Have intangible costs and benefits been appropriately included?
8. Have any outcomes been counted more than once?
9. How have the outcomes been valued?
10. Have calculations for NPV of all options been appropriately performed?
11. Have appropriate sensitivity analyses been conducted?
12. Have sensitivity analyses been conducted for intangible benefits and costs?
13. Does the presentation of results include appropriate information?
    a. Are results presented in terms of NPV and not as cost-benefit ratios?
    b. Are techniques used to estimate intangibles clearly identified?

c. Are results presented in a way that clearly outlines to decision makers what options have been evaluated and how robust the CBA can be considered?

REFERENCES

1. Dupuit J. On the measurement of utility of public works. *Int Economic Papers* 1952;2:83–110.
2. Petty W. *Political arithmetick, or a discourse concerning the extent and value of land, people, buildings, etc.* London: Robert Caluel, 1699.
3. Rice D. *Estimating the cost of illness.* DHEW, PHS, 1966: Health Economics Series No. 6.
4. Weisbrod B. Costs and benefits of medical research. *J Political Economy* 1971;79:527–44.
5. Grosse R. Cost-benefit analysis of health services. *Ann Am Acad Political Soc Sci* 1972;89:399–418.
6. Klarman H. Application of cost-benefit analysis to the health services and a special case of technological innovation. *Soc Sci Med* 1975;4:325–44.
7. Dunlop D. Benefit-cost analysis: a review of its applicability in policy analysis for delivering health services. *Soc Sci Med* 1975;9:133–51.
8. Pauker S, Kassirer J. Therapeutic decision making: a cost-benefit analysis. *N Engl J Med* 1975;293:229–38.
9. Harrington W, Portney PR. Valuing the benefits of health and safety regulation. *J Urban Economics* 1987;22:101–12.
10. Thompson MS. Willingness to pay and accept risks to cure chronic disease. *Am J Public Health* 1986;76:392–96.
11. Johannesson M. Economic evaluation of hypertension treatment. *Int J Technology Assessment in Health Care* 1992;8:506–23.
12. Fisher A, Chestnut LG, Violette DM. The value of reducing risks of death: a note on new evidence. *J Policy Analysis and Management* 1989;8(1):88–100.

BIBLIOGRAPHY

Berwick DM, Weinstein MC. What do patients value? Willingness to pay for ultrasound in normal pregnancy. *Med Care* 1985;23(7):881–93.
Estaugh SR. *Financing health care: economic efficiency and equity.* Dover, MA.: Auburn House Publishing Co., 1987.
Fuchs V, Zeckhauser R. Valuing health—a "priceless" commodity. *Am Econ Rev* 1987;77(2):263–68.
Ginsberg GM, Tulchinsky TH. Costs and benefits of a measles inoculation of children in Israel, the West Bank, and Gaza. *J Epidemiol Commun Health* 1990;44:272–80.
Hammond PB, Coppock R (eds). *Valuing health risks, costs, and benefits for environmental decision making: report of a conference.* Washington, D.C.: National Academy Press, 1990.
Health care cost-benefit and cost-effectiveness analysis (CBA/CEA) from 1979 to 1990: a bibliography. *Med Care* 1993;31(7): supplement (July)JS1–JS150.

Johannesson M, Jonsson B. Economic evaluation in health care: is there a role for cost-benefit analysis? *Health Policy* 1991;17:1–23.

Phelps C, Mushlin A. On the (near) equivalence of cost-effectiveness and cost-benefit analyses. *Int J Technology Assessment in Health Care* 1991;7(1):12–21.

Ponnighaus JM. The cost/benefit of measles immunization: a study from southern Zambia. *J Trop Med Hyg* 1980;83:141–49.

Udvarhelyi IS, Colditz GA, Rai A, Epstein AM. Cost-effectiveness and cost-benefit analyses in the medical literature; are the methods being used correctly? *Ann Intern Med* 1992;116:238–44.

8

Cost-Effectiveness Analysis

ANNE C. HADDIX
PHAEDRA A. SHAFFER

This chapter focuses on specific aspects of cost-effectiveness analysis (CEA) and provides guidance on when to use CEA, how to frame CEA study questions, and how to value costs of disease averted for CEA. Determining the cost of disease using the cost-of-illness approach constitutes a major portion of this chapter, since this component of the net cost is critical to CEA. This chapter is not intended to stand alone as a guide for performing CEA; rather, it summarizes the techniques described throughout this book, highlighting recommendations specific for CEA.

DEFINITION OF COST-EFFECTIVENESS ANALYSIS

Cost-effectiveness analysis is commonly used to conduct economic analyses of health programs.[1-3] In CEA, no attempt is made to assign a monetary value to disease averted beyond the cost of care for persons with these conditions and costs associated with lost productivity relating to morbidity and mortality. Rather, results are presented in the form of cost per health outcome, such as "cost per case prevented" or "cost per life saved." The decision maker is left to make value judgments about the intrinsic value of the health outcomes.

Cost-effectiveness analysis is most useful when the goal of the analysis is to identify the most cost-effective prevention strategy from a set of options that produce a common effect. Because CEA does not use a common outcome measure such as dollars or quality-adjusted life years (QALYs), it does not provide a convenient way to compare the cost-effectiveness of interventions for different health conditions. Another disadvantage is that judgments about the value and quality of lives must be implicitly made by the user of the study results because they are not included explicitly in a CEA.

BACKGROUND OF CEA

The use of CEA in health care began in the mid-1970s in response to a need for systematic analysis of health care decisions,[1,3] although those primarily of a clinical nature.[4-6] Cost-benefit analysis was considered too burdensome, and because of controversies over the valuation of health and life, it had fallen from favor. Health practitioners sought a less complex method in which the results were explicitly stated in terms of health outcomes rather than dollars.

The U. S. government began to use CEA in the late 1970s for public health decisions, particularly in vaccine policy.[7] Since then, CEA has become the predominate method for analyzing health-care decisions in both the clinical and public health sectors.

WHEN TO CONDUCT A CEA

CEA compares the costs of optional interventions or treatments per health outcome achieved. CEA is most useful when the interventions being compared have one clear and specific outcome. Four scenarios for which CEA is most suited include the following[8]:

1. Comparing alternative strategies for an identical goal
2. Identifying which intervention method is best for a specific population
3. Providing empirical support for the adoption of previously underfunded programs with low cost-effectiveness ratios
4. Identifying practices that are not worth their cost

HOW TO CONDUCT A CEA

Once CEA has been selected as the method of analysis, there are nine basic steps to conducting a CEA:

- Frame the problem to be analyzed
- Identify the options to be compared
- Identify the outcome measures
- Identify intervention and outcome costs
- Construct the decision tree
- Identify the probabilities
- Analyze the decision tree
- Perform sensitivity analysis
- Prepare presentation of results

Framing the Problem

The first step in CEA actually has several components, all of which need to be carefully considered to assure that the study will be productive and useful. A detailed description of components in framing the problem is provided in chapter 2; the following sections summarize some highlights related to CEA.

The study question and the scope of the evaluation must be defined. The study question determines which interventions should be included in the study and helps define the scope of the analysis. Defining the scope of the analysis involves specifying the economic perspective, the time frame of the analysis, and the analytic horizon. The perspective describes the costs and consequences that will be included in the analysis and indicates whether they will be included in the numerator or denominator of the summary measure. The time frame delineates the capture period of the intervention, and the analytic horizon indicates which future costs and benefits will be included. Each of these components, with specific attention to cost-effectiveness analysis, is discussed in greater detail below.

Study Question

As discussed in chapter 2, a clearly stated study question will make conducting a CEA much easier by eliminating false starts. By focusing and reducing complexity, a good study question will make the results more useful to decision makers. The scope of the analysis should flow logically from the study question; if the scope does not flow logically, the study question should be reexamined.

Some examples of questions that could be answered through CEA include:

- Which drug is the most cost-effective for treating persons with *Chlamydia* infection?
- Which tobacco-control program is most cost-effective in the Southeast Asian community?
- Are needle-exchange programs more cost-effective than HIV-awareness programs among intravenous drug users?
- Is surgical treatment of patients with prostate cancer cost-effective?

Perspective

Once the interventions have been identified, the perspective must be defined. To do this, the researcher must answer the question, "Who is responsible for the costs and consequences of the programs being evaluated?" For example, will society as a whole, the federal government, a state government, an employer, a private health insurer, or an individual be responsible for the costs and consequences of the program? An economic evaluation could take the perspective of any of these entities or of some other relevant entity.

Adopting a particular perspective may require measuring different costs and consequences or including costs differently in the summary measures. The following example shows how changing the perspective of a study to measure the cost of blindness results in the inclusion of different costs. If the study were conducted from the perspective of a private health-care provider, only the costs associated with the provision of care would be included. If this narrow perspective were used to set policy on a national scale, public health resources might be allocated inefficiently. If the perspective were changed to that of society, additional costs (e.g., the earnings forgone because of disability, the cost of retraining, and the cost of special equipment for the seeing-impaired) would be included. The broader perspective is frequently more useful because the resulting policies will maximize the efficiency of health-care spending for the whole population.

For this reason, economic analyses typically use the societal perspective. This approach includes all costs regardless of who pays and who benefits.

> *Recommendation:* All cost-effectiveness analyses should take the societal perspective. Additional perspectives may also be taken when relevant to the study question. The perspectives of the analysis should be clearly stated in the presentation of the study.

Time Frame

The second step in defining the scope of the study is determining the time frame and the analytic horizon for the analysis (see "Analytic Horizon" below). The time frame should correspond to the time period in which the intervention costs will occur. Specifically, the time frame of the study should include the time period in which the intervention or treatment is delivered. The time frame should extend long enough to ensure that relevant consequences of the intervention are captured. For example, a study looking for improvement in birth outcomes as a result of a prenatal nutrition program should have a time frame of at least 9 months.

In many cases, a 1-year time frame is the most practical. Data from health-care facilities, such as the number of tests or persons participating in a program, are often available for a calendar month or for a fiscal year. Using data from a full year eliminates any seasonal variation in participation. A multiyear time frame may be more appropriate for interventions with extended start-up time, high initial cost, or long treatment period.

> *Recommendation:* The time frame must be long enough to capture relevant outcomes. When practical, a 1-year time frame should be used. Longer time frames should be used for interventions with extended start-up time, high initial costs, or long intervention periods over which effectiveness may vary.

In multiyear evaluations, the *present value* of costs and monetary benefits are *discounted* to the base year of the analysis, as discussed in chapter 6. The cost of disease averted after the first year should also be discounted. Discounting is a method for adjusting the value of future costs and benefits. Discounting (expressed as the present value of a dollar) is based on the time value of money, which means that a dollar received today is worth more than the same dollar received in the future. This is true even if inflation is not considered, since a dollar received now can be invested and earn interest.

Discounting of costs and monetary benefits is required in CEA. Discounting of nonmonetary benefits is more controversial, since no consensus exists that a year of good health now is more valuable than a year of good health in the future. In general, discounting of nonmonetary benefits is recommended to maintain constant cost-effectiveness ratios across years. A more detailed presentation of discounting and other time adjustment issues, including the selection of a discount rate and the calculation of net present values, is presented in chapter 5.

Recommendation: Future monetary and nonmonetary costs and benefits should be discounted at either 3% or 5%, with sensitivity analyses performed using 0% and 8%.

Analytic Horizon

Although in most cases, the time frame for the study will be at least 1 year, the analytic horizon may be longer. The analytic horizon is the entire period over which benefits can be realized or costs incurred. The analytic horizon may be the lifetime of an individual who received the intervention during the time frame of the study. In the prenatal nutrition example above, the time frame was 1 year; however, the benefits of improved birth outcomes might extend well beyond that year. It is important to remember that future costs and benefits must be discounted in order to reflect accurately the time value of money.

Recommendation: The analytic horizon should be long enough to capture all benefits and costs that occur in the future as a result of the program. These costs and benefits should be discounted at either 3% or 5%, with sensitivity analysis using 0% and 8%.

Identification of Interventions

Once the problem to be analyzed has been structured, the next step is to identify the interventions to be compared. The choice of interventions is very important. A cost-effectiveness analysis can be done very precisely, but if it does not evaluate all relevant interventions, it will not be useful.

When selecting interventions, all reasonable options, subject to the constraints indicated below, should be included. Interventions must be appropriate for the target population. Measures of effectiveness for the intervention must exist. The intervention must be legally, morally, and ethically acceptable to policymakers and society. Finally, it is important to remember that CEA must compare options that are directed at achieving the same health outcome.

The set of options should always include current practice. Current practice may include the "no-program" option. The current practice option serves as a reference or baseline. The current practice alternative is included in the model, regardless of a priori decisions about its continued use, so an incremental cost for all new interventions under consideration can be derived.

Recommendation: The list of alternative intervention strategies in a CEA should include all reasonable options and a baseline comparator (usually either the current practice or no program).

Identify Outcome Measures

In a CEA, components of the measure of health outcome appear in both the numerator and the denominator. The costs of disease that is averted as a result of the intervention appear in the net-cost calculation that comprises the numerator. The direct measure of the health outcomes prevented (e.g., cases prevented, lives saved) is the denominator of the CEA ratio. This section discusses the selection of the appropriate health outcome measure for a CEA.

The health outcome identified for the study must be relevant to address the study question, and the outcome must be the same for each intervention. A health outcome often used in CEA is life years saved. Other commonly used outcome measures include lives saved, cases prevented, and cases identified.

Intermediate and Final Outcomes

There are two basic categories of health outcomes: intermediate and final. Intermediate outcomes are often those most directly associated with the intervention being evaluated. Examples of intermediate outcomes include cases identified or behavior changed. Measures of intermediate outcomes do not attempt to establish the relationship between intervention and final outcome. Intermediate-outcome measures should only be used when the relationship between the intermediate- and final-outcome measure is not known.

Final-outcome measures include cases prevented, lives saved, deaths averted, and life years gained. Final-outcome measures may be direct measures of an intervention or may be derived from the intermediate outcomes if the relationship between the intermediate outcome and final outcome is known.

Consider a CEA that examines different interventions for reducing blood-lead levels in children. In this case, the intermediate outcome that is a direct effect of the program is a health outcome—i.e., the number of children with blood-lead levels of less than 10 μg/dl. The final outcome measure may be in terms of IQ points gained. Unfortunately, because the relationship between blood-lead levels and IQ has not been definitively established, a final-outcome measure is not available. In this case, the intermediate-outcome measure is often used.

It is recommended that, when they exist, final-outcome measures be used in cost-effectiveness analysis. When intermediate-outcome measures are used, the limitations that prevent the use of a final-outcome measure should be discussed in the presentation of the study.

> *Recommendation:* Final health-outcome measures should be used in CEA, unless the relationship between the intermediate outcomes and the final health outcome is not known.

Adverse Effects of an Intervention

In addition to the health outcomes an intervention is designed to prevent, the intervention itself may also cause harmful side effects or adverse health effects. For example, many types of antibiotic therapy are associated with gastrointestinal disorders. This side effect may result in additional treatment costs that should be factored into the analysis. Minor side effects that do not ultimately change the structure of the decision model can be accounted for in terms of the additional cost they add to the intervention.

If there are serious adverse effects from the intervention, these should appear explicitly in the decision model as an outcome at a terminal node or through changes in the tree structure or the probabilities at the chance nodes. If the adverse effects are severe enough to warrant discontinuing therapy, the probability for treatment compliance should reflect this. Additional outcomes also may be needed to account for the adverse effects. For example, a decision analysis of strategies to increase folic acid intake for women of child-bearing age in an effort to prevent neural tube defects evaluated the cost-effectiveness of fortifying all cereal grains. However, an increase in folic acid intake by older persons may complicate the diagnosis of vitamin B12 deficiency and may ultimately result in permanent neurologic complications and death. Because of the serious nature of these adverse effects, the model included the outcomes of delayed diagnosis of vitamin B12 deficiency.[9]

The costs of disease in a CEA, whether a desired or an adverse effect, are determined using the same method, the cost-of-illness approach. This method is discussed in the next section.

Identify Intervention and Outcome Costs

Once the set of relevant intervention strategies and the health outcomes have been identified, the next step is to determine the costs of the components in the net cost equation:[10]

$$\text{Net Cost} = \text{Cost}_{\text{Intervention}} - \text{Cost}_{\text{DiseaseAverted}} - \text{Cost}_{\text{ProductivityLossesAverted}}$$

Net costs are divided into the total costs for all resources required for the program ($\text{Cost}_{\text{Intervention}}$), including the cost of side effects and the costs to participants, the costs of diagnosis and treatment associated with cases of the health problem averted ($\text{Cost}_{\text{Disease Averted}}$), and the productivity losses averted as a result of the intervention ($\text{Cost}_{\text{ProductivityLossesAverted}}$).

The costs of the optional intervention can be ascertained by following the guidelines given in chapter 5. In CEA, the costs of the disease averted and the productivity losses are assessed using the cost-of-illness approach. A description of this method is included below.

Illness and injuries place a large burden on society. The costs of these conditions include the costs of medical care and other nonmedical expenses, loss of productivity and leisure activities, grief, pain, and suffering. Prevention aims to reduce these costs. This section describes methods for assessing the economic cost of disease averted in CEA. These methods are also used to assess the costs of side effects of an intervention.

Willingness-to-Pay and Cost-of-Illness Defined

Two basic approaches to assessing the economic cost of disease are (1) the willingness-to-pay (WTP) method, and (2) the cost-of-illness (COI) method. The WTP method estimates the cost of an injury or disease by calculating what society would be willing to pay to avoid or reduce the likelihood of the injury or disease (see chapter 7). The COI method[11-17] estimates (1) the direct medical costs, (2) the direct nonmedical costs, and (3) the indirect costs of lost productivity associated with morbidity or premature mortality resulting from the health problem.

Although both the WTP and COI approaches for assessing the economic costs of disease have strengths and weaknesses (see Table 7.1), the COI method is most often used to measure the cost of disease in a CEA or a CUA. The WTP method is a more comprehensive measure than the COI and is often the method used to assess the economic costs of a health outcome in a CBA. Since the COI approach is the appropriate method for assessing the cost of disease averted, including productivity losses averted, in CEAs, this section focuses only on the COI method. For more information on the WTP approach, see chapter 7 on CBA.

Recommendation: The willingness-to-pay method or another comprehensive measure should be used to value health outcomes for CBAs. The cost-of-illness approach should be limited to estimating the cost of disease averted in CEA and CUAs.

The COI has two components: medical and nonmedical costs and productivity losses. Table 8.1 categorizes types of costs, which are discussed below.

Medical and Nonmedical Costs

The first component of costs calculated in the COI approach includes direct medical and nonmedical costs. *Medical costs* are the costs incurred to secure medical treatment and medications. Examples of medical costs include the cost of hospitalization, diagnostic testing, prescription drugs, and visits to a clinician. *Nonmedical costs* are the costs that are incurred in connection with medical treatment but that are not expended for medical treatment itself. An example of a nonmedical cost would be the cost of transportation (e.g., to visit a clinician) associated with the health problem. The categories of costs are created to allow disaggregation by the perspective taken. For example, only medical costs would be included in an analysis that takes the health-care-system perspective.

Prevalence- and Incidence-Based Costs

Prevalence-based costs are the total costs associated with the *existing* cases of a health problem that accrue in a specific period, divided by the total population. Prevalence-based costs estimate the value of resources lost during a specific period as the result of a health condition, regardless of when the condition became evident. Thus, in a prevalence-based prevention-effectiveness study with a time frame of 1 year, all cases of a health problem would be counted (including both new and existing cases); however, *only* costs of those cases incurred during the 1-year period would be counted.

Prevalence-based costs are useful in prevention-effectiveness studies of health problems of short duration. If the duration of the health problem does not extend beyond the period of the intervention, prevalence-based estimates can be used.

Prevalence-based costs are more commonly found in the literature and are

Table 8.1 Examples of Costs

DIRECT COSTS	DIRECT COSTS (*Continued*)	DIRECT COSTS (*Continued*)

Institutional inpatient care
  terminal care
  hospice
  hospitalization specialized
    units (e.g., ICU,
    CCU)
  nursing home
Institutional outpatient services
  clinic
  HMO
  emergency room
Home health care
Physician services
  primary care physicians
  medical specialists
  psychiatrists
Ancillary services
  psychologists
  social workers
  nutritionist
  physical and occupational
    therapy
  ambulance
  volunteer
Overhead allocated to tech-
    nology
  fixed costs of utilities
  space
  storage
  support services: laundry,
    housekeeping, admin-
    istration
  capital costs (depreciated
    over life of equipment)
    construction of facilities
  relocation expenses
  device or equipment cost
Variable costs of utilities
Medications (prescription and
  nonprescription)
  drug costs
  treating side effects or tox-
    icity of medications
  prophylaxis of side effects
  ordering and inventorying
  preparation
  training in new procedures
  dispensing and administra-
    tion
  monitoring
Devices and appliances
  prostheses
  glasses
  hearing aids
  ostomy supplies
  hypodermic needles
	home urine and blood-
	    testing equipment
	  ordering and inventorying
	Drugs, supplies, devices pro-
	    vided by household
	Research and development:
	  basic and applied
	  research
	Diagnostic tests
	  community screening pro-
	    gram
	  consumable supplies, per-
	    sonnel time, equip-
	    ment
	  imaging
	  laboratory testing
	  costs of false-positive and
	    false-negative cases
	  treating sequelae of unde-
	    tected disease
	Treatment services
	  surgery, initial and repeat
	  recovery room
	  anesthesia services
	  pathology services
	  acquisition costs for organ
	    transplants
	  consumable supplies, per-
	    sonnel, time, equip-
	    ment
	  treatment of complications
	  blood products
	  oxygen
	  radiation therapy
	  special diets
	Prevention services
	  screening space
	  vaccination, prophylaxis
	  disease prevention in
	    contacts of known
	    cases
	Rehabilitation
	Training and education
	  health education
	  self-care training for patients
	  life support skills for general
	    population
	  public awareness programs
	Care provided by family and
	    friends
	Transportation to and from
	    medical services
	Child care
	Housekeeping
	Modification of home to ac-
	    commodate patient
		Social services
		  family counseling
		  retraining, reeducation
		  sheltered workshops
		  employment services
		Program evaluation
		  monitoring impact of pro-
		    gram or technology
		  data analysis
		Repair of property destruction
		  (alcoholism, psychiatric
		  illness drug addiction)
		Law enforcement costs
		
		INDIRECT COSTS
		
		*Wages/Time**
		Change in productivity result-
		  ing from change in
		  health status
		  morbidity
		  mortality
		  averted illness
		Lost productivity while on the
		  job
		  absenteeism
		Income lost by family members
		Forgone leisure time
		Time spent by patient seeking
		  medical services
		Time spent by family and
		  friends attending pa-
		  tient (e.g., hospital vis-
		  itations)
		Intangible
		Psychosocial costs
		  apprehension, anxiety
		  grief and loss of well-being
		    associated with:
		    impending death
		    disfigurement
		    disability
		    economic and physical de-
		      pendence
		    loss of job
		    loss of opportunity for pro-
		      motion and education
		    social isolation
		    family conflict
		Valuations others put on pa-
		  tient's health and well-
		  being
		Pain
		Changes is social functioning
		  and activities of daily
		  living

*Quantifiable in monetary terms

Source: Reprinted with permission of Cambridge University Press from Luce BR and Elixhauser A. (1990). Int J of Technology Assessment in Health Care, Vol. 6.

frequently reported as annual costs of a health problem. If the problem does not extend beyond a 1-year period, the total cost of the health problem can be divided by the number of cases to obtain a cost per case of that health problem, which can be used in CEA. Care must be taken when attempting to convert prevalence-based costs of health problems with longer durations to incidence-based estimates.

Incidence-based costs are the total lifetime costs resulting from disease or illness. Prevention-effectiveness studies include incidence-based costs of new cases of a health problem that occur within the time frame of the analysis or occur as the result of an exposure during the time frame of the analysis.

Incidence-based costs include the medical care that is required for the duration of the illness, other costs associated with the illness, and lifetime productivity losses, measured as lost earnings, the result from morbidity or mortality related to the health condition. Since incidence-based costs often include costs that will occur in the future, discounting is performed to convert future costs to their present value in the base year of analysis.

Although incidence-based costs are more useful for policymaking situations, they are more difficult to obtain. Because lifetime costs are considered, incidence-based costs require knowledge of the course and duration of the health problem and the disabling impact of the problem and its chronic sequelae on employment and earnings over the lifetime of an individual.

> *Recommendation:* Incidence-based cost estimates of health outcomes should be used in CEA and CUA of prevention interventions unless the health problem being considered is of sufficiently short duration that prevalence-based estimates are equivalent to incidence-based estimates.

In calculating incidence-based costs, the first step is to review the literature to determine whether reliable incidence-based estimates of the health outcome exist. If none are available, and no prevalence-based costs exist which may be transformed to incidence-based estimates, the next step is to develop an itemized list of all medical services (e.g., hospital days, number of visits to clinicians, pharmaceuticals) necessary to treat the person for the health problem. If treatment varies extremely from case to case, it may be useful to categorize cases. For example, in cost-of-illness studies of food-borne illness, cases are often classified as mild (no visits to a clinician), moderate (outpatient visits to a clinician), and severe (requiring hospitalization). If the treatment costs are complex or if they extend over a long period, costs may also be divided or calculated by stage of disease. An excellent example of an incidence-based cost-of-illness study is the article by Guinan, Farnham, and Holtgrave estimating the value of preventing an HIV infection.[18] A comprehensive list of costs found in cost-of-illness analyses is shown in Table 8.1.

Costs vs. Charges

When collecting medical costs, care should be taken to differentiate true economic *costs* from *charges*. True economic costs can be described as the value of forgone opportunities. If resources are used for one opportunity such as a cholesterol-screening program, those resources are no longer available for another public health program. The cost of the chosen option represents the opportunity cost of the option that was not chosen.

In a perfect marketplace, the charge or price for goods represents true economic cost. In the health-care arena, the charge (or price) of a product or service does not generally represent the true economic cost of that product or service. The medical marketplace is not an efficient market for two reasons.[19] First, a "list price," or charge, for a medical good or service may not represent the true economic cost of that good or service. List prices are greatly influenced by the involvement of government (i.e., Medicare and Medicaid), and several large third-party payers (e.g., large insurers, health maintenance organizations), which, because of their size and financial power base, may pay or negotiate discounted prices. Some suppliers of medical services may respond by instituting list prices that substantially inflate the true economic cost of goods or services in order to be compensated fully for the goods and services provided even when discounted payments are received. Self-payers and smaller insurance companies that are not able to negotiate discounts pay the higher list prices for the goods or services. Thus large discrepancies may exist among charges paid by large insurers, small insurers, and self-insurers.

The second reason for the discrepancy between costs and charges is that, in the health-care setting, some services and goods provided are profitable and some are not. Hence, providers often redistribute charges from less lucrative services to more lucrative services in order to make a profit. The result is that charges or financial (accounting) "costs" of a product or service may bear little resemblance to true economic costs. In addition, individual hospital bills may include charges for services outside the standard course of treatment. For example, a hospital bill for maternity services for a particular individual might include charges for a sterilization procedure. Inclusion of the unrelated sterilization procedure would distort the cost of service described as "maternity."

Health care providers often shift costs from uninsured patients to insured patients to recover costs for unreimbursed medical services. All patients are charged for medical services at a rate above the actual cost to recover costs from that portion of the patient population that does not pay—or fully pay—for health care received.

Thus charges for medical goods and services frequently do not reflect the actual resource costs. With the distinction between costs and charges in mind, it is recommended that true economic costs be determined when possible.

Recommendation: Resource costs rather than charges should be obtained when possible for prevention-effectiveness studies.

Collecting Cost Data
Sources for collecting cost data include the following:

Medicare Reimbursement Data. Since the government is afforded a "discount" of the health-care charges, its reimbursement data will more accurately reflect true economic costs than costs paid by small insurance companies or self-payers. However, Medicare reimbursement data are only specific to the elderly population and therefore may not represent societal costs in general. Medicare reimbursement data can be obtained from individual states or at the national level through such sources as *The DRG Handbook* (see Appendix E).

Blue Cross/Blue Shield Data. This organization provides data on its reimbursement for services. Blue Cross/Blue Shield breaks down medical services into small units and determines the amount of money that it will reimburse for each unit of medical service. Because the charges are listed separately, it may be easier to determine true economic cost for an injury or disease. Appendix E provides additional information on securing these data.

Charges Obtained from Hospital Records. This information can be converted to cost data by using Medicare conversion rates published in the *Federal Register.* The *Federal Register* publishes these conversion rates on a state-by-state basis each year, for both urban and rural populations. See Appendix F for current conversion rates by state.

Physician Visits and Charges. Data on costs and the number of visits to physicians stratified by age group can be found in the most recent edition of the *Statistical Abstract of the U.S.*[20] Costs can be updated, if necessary, using the medical component of the Consumer Price Index (CPI) in Appendix G. These data are what is actually paid per visit to a physician, and therefore will more closely represent true economic costs.

Panel of Experts. Such a group can be asked to estimate procedure costs. However, this method may yield an extremely broad range of results and is based on subjective judgment.

Data on medical and nonmedical costs are available from several sources. Appendix E provides a list and description of several widely used sources that include literature indexes, public use tapes, annually published materials, and contractual services. For example, a 1993 supplement to *Medical Care* provides an excellent source of cost-effectiveness and cost-benefit literature published in 1979–1990 and related to specific illnesses.[21]

If, however, cost information cannot be obtained from the literature or the other data sources specified in Appendix E, it may be possible to collect information directly from the source of the intervention. For example, if data are needed on medical costs for screening for gonorrhea, a clinic that does such screening might provide cost data related to cost of treatment, cost of tests, and cost of labor involved for the intervention.

Adjustments to Cost Data
When COI estimates have been determined for a year prior to the base year of the economic evaluation, cost estimates should be inflated to base-year dollars, assuming, of course, the services were similar in the two periods. Care should

also be taken to ensure that cost estimates obtained from the existing literature are also adjusted to the base year. Appendix H provides the Consumer Price Index by major medical categories, e.g., medical care, medical-care services (which includes professional services and hospital rooms), and medical-care commodities for the period 1960–1994, which can be used to make adjustments for inflation. Chapter 6 provides a more detailed explanation of accounting for the time differential of money, including how to use the CPI to inflate dollars to the base year of the study.

As mentioned earlier, COI estimates converted to base-year dollars enter the economic analysis in the year in which the health problem occurs. To determine total net lifetime cost of illness, an estimate of the present value of lifetime cost of illness is used. This estimate is then discounted to reflect a net present value for the stream of future costs. Discounting methods and values are discussed in chapter 6.

Productivity Losses and Intangible Costs
In addition to medical and nonmedical costs, two other types of costs can be considered when assessing the economic costs of a health outcome: productivity losses and intangible costs. Whereas medical and nonmedical costs are described as "resources expended," productivity losses can be described as "resources forgone." Productivity losses attempt to measure the economic burden an illness places upon an individual.

Productivity losses associated with a health problem are the patient- or caregiver-borne costs resulting from unnecessary morbidity and premature mortality. These are costs that must be included when undertaking a study from a societal perspective, because they are costs to society as a whole (society's costs related to reduced levels of output, time spent to obtain health care, and lost productivity resulting from some change in employment status as a result of morbidity or mortality). If cases of the adverse health condition can be averted, the morbidity, mortality, and costs associated with that health condition can also be averted.

The COI method of evaluating the cost of a disease estimates only medical and nonmedical costs and productivity losses, and does not include the costs associated with pain and suffering. *Intangible costs* represent costs for pain and suffering and other costs for which a monetary value cannot be easily assigned. Because COI does not account for pain and suffering and does not fully capture the economic value of reducing the risk of developing a disease, the COI method does not completely measure the benefits of an intervention and is not generally used in a cost-benefit analysis. Therefore the WTP method is the preferred approach to use in a cost-benefit analysis.

The human-capital (HC) method, developed by Rice and others,[11–15,22] is used to assess the productivity losses from illness or injury, as measured by income forgone because of morbidity or mortality. Labor force participation rates and earnings of affected persons are used to calculate the value of productivity lost because of morbidity or premature mortality. Thus the value of productivity losses from an individual's disability or death is based on an estimate of the present value of the individual's future income stream. As discussed earlier in this chapter, productivity losses associated with time lost from work to participate in an intervention program or as the result of morbidity from side effects of an intervention can also be calculated by the HC method.

The HC approach for assessing productivity losses associated with a health outcome is not ideal.[14,22] The HC approach excludes the costs associated with pain and suffering, it values earnings and housekeeping services but not leisure time, and it may undervalue the productivity of groups whose productivity value is not reflected in earnings, e.g., volunteer workers. The category of earnings measures the value of employment but does not fully measure an individual's contribution to society. Also, some groups may be valued more highly than others when only wages are considered. Males may be valued more highly than females, for example, because males typically receive higher wages than females for the same job. And younger, working individuals would be valued more highly than older, retired persons.

Some questions have been raised about the appropriateness of attempts to assign a monetary value to human life.[22] This argument is used to oppose the inclusion of productivity losses in cost-effectiveness studies, regardless of whether the HC or other valuation approaches are used. However, taken in context, the HC approach attempts to calculate only the economic burden of illness and does not attempt to assign a value to a human life or to the pain and suffering associated with a health problem. Bearing this in mind, the HC estimation of mortality costs associated with a health problem should be considered the lower-bound estimate of the economic cost of mortality. It should also be noted that the WTP approach does not attempt to place a value on a human life but on the value an individual or society places on reducing the risk of death.

Recommendation: The human-capital approach should be used to estimate productivity losses for CEA.

Morbidity Costs

Morbidity costs can be defined as the wages lost by people who are unable to work or perform normal housekeeping duties because of a health problem they have or one experienced by another individual for whom they must care, e.g., a child or elderly parent.[15] The total cost of morbidity is determined by the number of days sick or hospitalized (and the number of days required by a care giver), multiplied by the daily wage rate. Daily wages can be used as an approximation for lost productivity. Unless data are available, assumptions can be made as to the number of recuperation days required per hospital day. For example, for every 1 day in the hospital, one might assume that 1 to 2 days of at-home recuperation are needed, depending on the severity of the illness. For instances in which there are insufficient data on the cost variables, a range of estimates should be used.

The daily wage rate can be estimated using the *Average Weekly Earnings* published by the U. S. Department of Commerce, Bureau of Labor Statistics. If these data are used, fringe benefits, the value of housekeeping services, and the labor force participation rates may also need to be included. Appendix I, Table 1a, presents selected economic variables used in estimating annual earnings by age (in 1990 dollars), which in turn are used to calculate the costs of morbidity. Because the tables are arranged by age and sex, it is necessary to know the distribution by age and sex of the at-risk population being studied. However, if the distribution by age and sex is unknown, a mean value (weighted by age and sex) can be calculated to provide a value for average annual earnings (see below). When reporting results, a description of the age and sex distribution of the at-risk population should be included in the discussion.

The mean value of a lost work day is estimated at $94 in 1990 dollars. This is calculated by dividing the average annual earnings, $23,582, by 250 working days. If the days of morbidity reported do not distinguish between a work day or a nonwork day, the mean value of an unspecified day is estimated at $65, calculated by dividing the same average annual earnings by 365 days. Morbidity costs are updated to "years beyond 1990," using the increase in earnings reported annually in the *Employment and Earnings* March supplement, published by the U. S. Department of Commerce, Bureau of Labor Statistics. Chapter 6 explains this calculation. Table 1a in Appendix I also provides a summary of the assumptions for the above calculations. These data assume that the entire population has productive potential, thus allowing adaptation to a base year without taking the 1990 unemployment rate into account.

Mortality Costs

The cost of mortality using the HC approach is the future productivity lost to society as the result of premature death. This value is derived by estimating the present value (PV) of future earnings lost by an individual who dies prematurely.[15,22] As in the calculation of morbidity costs, the HC approach applies labor force participation rates and earnings to persons who die prematurely as a result of an adverse health outcome.

The economic variables, and their assumptions, used to calculate morbidity costs are the same variables and assumptions used to calculate mortality costs. Appendix I, Table 2, projects the present value of future lifetime earnings, by age, using the recommended discount rate of either 3% or 5%, as well as the range in rates from 0% to 10%. If the age distribution of the at-risk population is not known or if the analyst wishes to remove age and sex bias from the estimates, Table 2 also presents the mean present value of lifetime earnings for the U. S. population, weighted by age or sex.

When the recommended 5% discount rate is used, the mean present value of the expected future lifetime earnings for a person, regardless of age or sex, is $679,507 in 1990 dollars. The table provides a summary of the assumptions used in the above calculation. Estimates can be updated to years after 1990 using the method described for morbidity costs.

When assessing the costs of injury or disease averted, productivity losses should be presented separately from medical and nonmedical costs. The dollars saved on medical and nonmedical costs are fundamentally different from the dollars saved by preventing productivity losses. Cost information may be interpreted in different ways depending on the decision maker's need. For example, a decision maker may be specifically interested in the impact of an intervention of the health care system, in which case only direct medical and nonmedical costs (resources expended) should be included in the analysis. Therefore, it is recommended that two sets of results in a cost analysis be presented: (1) results that include direct medical and nonmedical costs only, and (2) results that include both direct medical and nonmedical costs and productivity losses.

Recommendations for using the cost-of-illness approach to valuing health outcomes in CEA and CUA are listed below.

Recommendation: The numerator of a CEA should be the net cost of an intervention. Thus the cost of the disease averted should appear in the net-cost equation.

Recommendation: The cost-of-illness method should be used to estimate the cost of disease averted in a CEA.

Recommendation: A CEA should be performed with only direct medical and nonmedical costs in the net-cost equation and, again, with the sum of direct medical and nonmedical costs and productivity losses. In the special case of a cost-utility analysis, only direct costs should be included in the net-cost calculation if the health outcome measure in the denominator accounts for changes in employment status (see chapter 9).

Constructing the Decision Tree

Now that the preparatory work has been done, a decision tree can be constructed. This may be the most critical step of the analysis. Constructing the tree is the process by which nodes are mapped out and values are assigned to them. This step is described in chapter 3. The focus of this section is the data requirements for using this analytic framework to conduct a CEA. A CEA uses a combination of epidemiologic and economic data. Unless the interventions being considered have been carefully evaluated by the decision team, the first step in data collection is usually a thorough literature review.

In the ideal analysis, data would be available from randomized, controlled trials or other well-designed studies that had undergone peer review and had been published in the scientific literature. Practically speaking, there are often gaps in the data that must be filled. One way that a gap can be filled is by designing a study to answer the relevant question. However, this is often not feasible because of time and resource constraints and is frequently unnecessary. Such gaps can also be filled by using expert panels to develop best estimates or by assigning values on the basis of available evidence. If these methods are used, the variables must be viewed as being uncertain and should be subjected to sensitivity analysis. Those that are critical to the results of the CEA may require additional study.

A list of basic types of data needed to construct a cost-effectiveness decision tree is provided in Table 8.2. However, every analysis is different, and some may require additional or different data.

Once the data have been collected, the tree itself can be constructed. Decision-analysis software is available (see Appendix B). Most software packages include cost-effectiveness analysis as an option.

The software program can then be used to analyze the dual scales (cost and health outcome) simultaneously in order to compute the expected total cost and the expected value of the health outcome for each strategy. The strategies are ranked in ascending or descending order of cost or effectiveness depending on software-user preference. The software will also compute the average and incremental cost-effectiveness ratios. These summary measures are defined and discussed below.

First, the measures of effectiveness and the risk associated variables are expressed as probabilities in the decision tree. Then, the costs and outcome variables are assigned as dual values of the terminal nodes. When conducting a CEA with decision software, the cost-effectiveness option allows the user to enter two sets of values for the terminal nodes in the model. The first set of values represents the costs, and the second set represents the health outcome. The total cost is the sum of the costs of all events that occur on the path to the terminal node. The effectiveness is entered as the health outcome of the terminal node. Health outcomes are entered either as a quantified health outcome, e.g., number of years of life or as a binomial count variable (e.g., 1 = case of disease; 0 = no case of disease). Figure 8.1 presents a complete decision tree for vaccination strategies for Disease XYZ in Appendix D, including the probabilities and dual outcomes.

Table 8.2 Data Needed to Construct a Cost-Effectiveness Decision Tree

1. Measurement of the effectiveness of an intervention
   * Efficacy of intervention
   * Compliance, participation, effectiveness in a community setting
   * Sensitivity and specificity of laboratory tests
   * Prevalence of risk factors

2. Risk of side effects

3. Risk of disease or injury with and without the intervention
   * Risk of primary disease or injury averted
   * Risk of sequelae or complications of disease or injury averted

4. Net cost of intervention
   * Medical and nonmedical costs of intervention program
   * Productivity losses in intervention program
   * Medical and nonmedical costs of side effects
   * Productivity losses from side effects
   * Medical and nonmedical costs of disease or injury, including the costs of sequelae or complications and productivity losses from morbidity and mortality

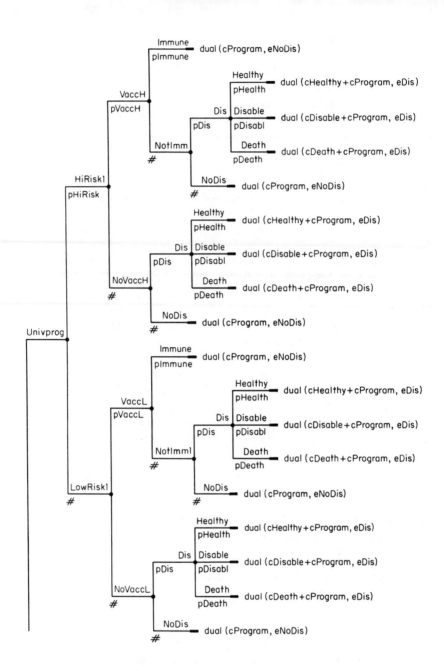

Figure 8.1 A complete decision tree for vaccination strategies for Disease XYZ using SMLTREE.

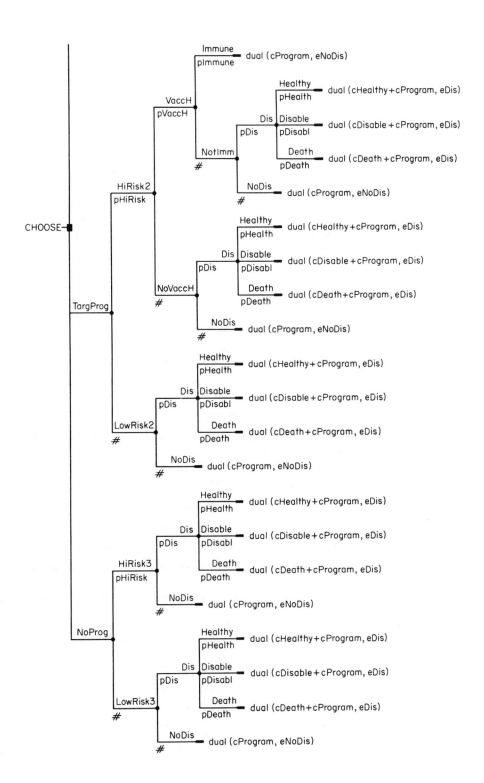

Analyzing the Tree and Interpreting the Results

Once values have been assigned to both the chance and terminal nodes, the branches are "averaged-out-and-folded-back" to produce expected values for both the costs and the outcomes of the options in the tree. These results are used to calculate both average and incremental cost-effectiveness (CE) ratios.

Average and Incremental Results

Generally, two types of CE ratios are reported for a CEA; the *average* CE ratio and the *incremental* CE ratio. Each provides insight into the efficiency and the affordability of the intervention. The average CE ratio, evaluated against the baseline or reference option, is the net cost of a strategy divided by the total number of health outcomes averted, e.g., cost per case prevented or year of life saved. The cost of the intervention in an average CE ratio is

$$\text{Intervention Cost} = \text{Cost}_{\text{InterventionA}}$$

where $\text{Cost}_{\text{InterventionA}}$ is the cost of the intervention for which the average CE ratio is calculated.

The second component of the numerator of the average CE ratio is the cost of the disease and productivity losses averted as a result of the intervention. The costs averted are

$$\text{Disease Cost Averted} = (\text{Cost}_{\text{Disease0}} + \text{Cost}_{\text{ProductivityLosses0}}) - (\text{Cost}_{\text{DiseaseA}} + \text{Cost}_{\text{ProductivityLossesA}})$$

Where $\text{Cost}_{\text{Disease0}} + \text{Cost}_{\text{ProductivityLosses0}}$ are the costs of the disease at the baseline state and $\text{Cost}_{\text{DiseaseA}} + \text{Cost}_{\text{ProductivityLossesA}}$ are the costs of the disease that still occur after the intervention is implemented.

The denominator of the average CE ratio is the total number of health outcomes prevented by the intervention

$$\text{Total Health Outcomes Prevented} = \text{Outcomes}_0 - \text{Outcomes}_A$$

where Outcomes_0 is the total number of outcomes that occur at the baseline and Outcomes_A is the total number of outcomes that occur after the intervention is implemented.

Based on the above, the formula for the average CE ratio for an intervention is

$$\text{Average CE Ratio} = \frac{(\text{Intervention Cost} - \text{Disease Cost Averted})}{\text{Total Health Outcomes Prevented}}$$

When the baseline is "no program," an alternative formula for calculating the average CE ratio which produces the same result can be used.

$$\text{Average CE ratio} = \frac{\text{Total Cost}_A - \text{Total Cost}_0)}{(\text{Total Outcomes}_0 - \text{Total Outcomes}_A)}$$

where *Total Cost* is sum of the cost of the intervention and the cost of the disease for each intervention and *Total Outcomes* is the total number of cases of disease that occur after each intervention is implemented. The two formulas are equivalent. Decision software, however, often reports CEAs as the total cost and total number of outcomes for each intervention. This formula was used to calculate the average CE ratios in Table 8.3.

The average CE ratio provides useful information about the overall affordability of an intervention. However, prevention-effectiveness studies are also used to examine the efficiency of one strategy relative to another. This is done by calculating incremental CE ratios. When intervention options are arrayed in order of increasing effectiveness, the incremental CE ratio is the difference in cost of any two adjacent options divided by the differences in number of health outcomes prevented by the two options. The incremental CE ratio is generally reported as the additional cost per additional health outcome prevented.

The cost of the intervention in an incremental CE ratio is

$$\text{Additional Intervention Cost} = \text{Cost}_{\text{InterventionB}} - \text{Cost}_{\text{InterventionA}}$$

where $\text{Cost}_{\text{InterventionB}}$ is the cost of the intervention for which the incremental CE ratio is calculated and $\text{Cost}_{\text{InterventionA}}$ is the cost of the next less effective intervention.

The second component of the numerator of the incremental CE ratio is the additional cost of the disease and productivity losses averted as a result of the intervention expressed as

$$\text{Additional Disease Cost Averted} = (\text{Cost}_{\text{DiseaseA}} + \text{Cost}_{\text{ProductivityLossesA}}) - (\text{Cost}_{\text{DiseaseB}} + \text{Cost}_{\text{ProductivityLossesB}})$$

where $\text{Cost}_{\text{DiseaseA}} + \text{Cost}_{\text{ProductivityLossesA}}$ are the costs of the disease at the adjacent option and $\text{Cost}_{\text{DiseaseB}} + \text{Cost}_{\text{ProductivityLossesB}}$ are the costs of the disease that still occur after the more effective intervention is implemented.

The denominator of the incremental CE ratio is the additional number of health outcomes prevented by the more effective intervention

$$\text{Additional Health Outcomes Prevented} = \text{Outcomes}_{\text{A}} - \text{Outcomes}_{\text{B}}$$

where $\text{Outcomes}_{\text{A}}$ is the total number of cases of disease that occur after implementation of the adjacent option and $\text{Outcomes}_{\text{B}}$ is the total number of cases of disease that occur after the more effective intervention is implemented.

Based on the above, the formula for the incremental CE ratio for an intervention is

$$\text{Incremental CE Ratio} = \frac{(\text{Additional Intervention Cost} - \text{Additional Disease Cost Averted})}{\text{Additional Health Outcomes Prevented}}$$

As with average CE ratios, an alternative formula for calculating the incremental CE ratio produces the same result

$$\text{Incremental CE ratio} = \frac{(\text{Total Cost}_{\text{B}} - \text{Total Cost}_{\text{A}})}{(\text{Total Outcomes}_{\text{A}} - \text{Total Outcomes}_{\text{B}})}$$

Table 8.3 Results of a Cost-Effectiveness Analysis: A Comparison of Average and Incremental Ratios

			Average Cost Effectiveness			Incremental Cost Effectiveness		
	Total Cost (billions)	Cases of Disease	Net Cost (Savings) (millions)[a]	Total Cases Prevented[a]	Average Cost (Savings) Per Case Prevented[b]	Additional Cost (Savings) (millions)[a]	Additional Cases Prevented[a]	Incremental Cost (Savings) Per Case Prevented[b]
No Program	$5.032	129,000						
Targeted Program	$4.206	105,250	($826)	23,750	($35,000)	($ 826)	23,750	($35,000)
Universal Program	$5.577	67,345	$545	61,655	$ 9,000	$1,371	37,905	$36,000

[a]Compared with no program
[b]Rounded to nearest thousand

where Total Cost is sum of the cost of each intervention and the cost of the disease that still occurs after the intervention is implemented and Total Outcomes is the total number of outcomes that occur after the intervention is implemented. The incremental CE ratios in Table 8.3 were calculated using this formula.

Incremental CE ratios are similar to but should not be confused with marginal CE ratios. Marginal CEA is the change in the cost-effectiveness as a result of expansion or contraction of an intervention. Often, a cost-effectiveness analysis is conducted in two stages. First, a marginal CEA is conducted to identify the most efficient size of each intervention. Then, an incremental CEA of different interventions is conducted in which the marginal CEA results are used to specify intervention efficiency and effectiveness.

Threshold Analysis

Although threshold analysis is often considered a type of sensitivity analysis, it may also be used to answer a specific policy question, and therefore the results of a threshold analysis would be reported with the average and incremental cost-effectiveness ratios. For example, a recent CEA of two drugs for treating patients for cervical *chlamydia* infection was designed to determine the price at which a more effective but more expensive drug could be subsituted for the less expensive but less effective drug with no change in total treatment costs. This price was determined by performing a threshold analysis on the price of the drug.[23]

Sensitivity Analysis

The final step in analyzing the model is to conduct sensitivity analyses on the variables that have uncertain values or that may change in different population settings. The types of strategies for sensitivity analysis are presented in chapter 3.

One advantage of using decision-analysis software is that the capacity for sensitivity analysis is built into these programs, and graphic displays of results are included. Sensitivity analyses are extremely important, because cost-effectiveness analysis is often conducted under conditions of uncertainty. The researcher must make assumptions about probabilities and costs when data are incomplete.

Sensitivity analyses should be performed on variables in the model for which uncertainty exists. By varying the value of a probability or cost systematically, sensitivity analysis makes it possible to identify the variables that have the greatest impact on the output of the model. This enables the researcher to identify research priorities. If changing the value of a variable about which there is a great deal of uncertainty has a substantial impact on the outcome of the model, a study can be designed to reduce uncertainty. However, if substantial changes in the value of an uncertain variable have little impact on the outcome, research resources might be better allocated elsewhere.

Multiple variables can be varied simultaneously, and their joint impacts can be evaluated. Most decision-analysis software has the capacity to present the results of sensitivity analyses graphically. Sensitivity analysis is a critical component of a cost-effectiveness analysis, and the results and their implications must be included in the presentation of the study.

Recommendation: Sensitivity analyses should be performed on all variables for which uncertainty exists, and the results should be included in the presentation of the study.

Table 8.4 presents the results of a "best-case"–"worst-case" sensitivity analysis for Disease XYZ. (See the Disease XYZ case study in Appendix D for interpretation of these results.)

Presentation of Results

A cost-effectiveness analysis with an elegant and sophisticated design is of little use if the results are not presented effectively. CEA is a tool for presenting information in a logical and clear way in order to assist in the decision-making process. Presentation is critical. The presentation of a cost-effectiveness analysis should include:

- The study perspective, time frame, and analytic horizon
- The study question
- The assumptions used to build the model
- A description of the interventions
- Evidence of the effectiveness of the interventions
- Identification of all relevant costs
    - Inclusion or exclusion of productivity costs
    - Discount rate
- Results of incremental analysis
- Results of sensitivity analysis
- Discussion of results that addresses all issues of concern and the implications of assumptions used

Table 8.4   Example of the Results of Sensitivity Analysis

	*Sensitivity Analysis: Incremental CE ratios**		
Perspective/ Strategy	*Best-Case Scenario*	*Base-Case Scenario*	*Worst-Case Scenario*
SOCIETAL			
Targeted	($37,000)	($35,000)	($32,000)
Universal	($3,000)	$36,000	$80,000
HEALTH CARE SYSTEM			
Targeted	($6,000)	($4,000)	($2,000)
Universal	$28,000	$67,000	$111,000

* Rounded to nearest thousand

So readers can gain a better sense of how this type of analysis is presented in the scientific literature, several cost-effectiveness articles are listed in the bibliography section for this chapter.

CONCLUSION

Cost-effectiveness analysis should be used to evaluate interventions that address a single and specific health outcome. Because no attempt is made to assign monetary values to health outcomes, cost-effectiveness analysis has been widely used in health evaluations. However, care must be taken when using the results of CEA. The results of CEA are most useful in, and should be limited to, evaluating multiple strategies to prevent a health problem.

This chapter has outlined the basic steps in conducting a CEA. The cost-of-illness approach to measuring the economic value of disease averted has been presented. Further reading material on the subject of CEA listed under Bibliography and the Disease XYZ case study presented in Appendix D will provide a supplement to the procedures described in this chapter.

REFERENCES

1. Weinstein MC, Stason WB. Foundations of cost-effectiveness for health and medical practices. *N Engl J Med* 1977;296:716–21.
2. Cohen DR, Henderson JB. *Health, prevention, and economics.* Oxford: Oxford Medical Publications, 1988.
3. Shepard DS, Thompson MS. First principles of cost-effectiveness analysis in health. *Public Health Rep* 1979;94:535–43.
4. McNeil BJ, Varady PD, Burrows BA et al. Measures of clinical efficacy: cost-effectiveness calculations in the diagnosis and treatment of hypertensive reno-vascular disease. *N Engl J Med* 1975;293:216–21.
5. Neuhauser D, Lewicki AM. What do we gain from the sixth stool guaiac? *N Engl J Med* 1975;293:226–28.
6. Weinstein M, Stasson W. Economic considerations in management of mild hypertension. Ann NY Acad Sci 1976;304:424–36.
7. U. S. Congress, Office of Technology Assessment. *A review of selected federal vaccine and immunization policies.* OTA-H-96. Washington, D.C.: Government Printing Office, 1979.
8. Emery DD, Schneiderman LJ. Cost-effectiveness analysis in health care. *Hastings Center Report* 1989; Jul–Aug:8–13.
9. Kelly AE, Scanlon KS, Mulinare J, Helmick CG, Haddix AC. Cost-effectiveness of alternative strategies to prevent neural tube defects in *Cost-effectiveness in Health and Medicine.* Gold MR, Siegel JE, Russell LB, Weinstein MC (eds.) New York: Oxford University Press, 1996.
10. Teutsch SM. A framework for assessing the effectiveness of disease and injury prevention. *MMWR* 1992;41 (No. RR-3):i–iv, 1–12.
11. Rice DP. *Estimating the cost of illness.* Health Economics Series, No. 6. Pub. No. 947-6. 1966. Washington, D.C.: U.S. Department of Health, Education, and Welfare.

12. Rice DP. Estimating the cost of illness. *Am J Public Health* 1967;57:424–40.
13. Rice DP, Cooper BS. The economic value of human life. *Am J Public Health* 1967; 57: 1954–66.
14. Rice DP, Hodgson TA. The value of human life revisited (editorial). *Am J Public Health* June 1982;72(6):536–38.
15. Rice DP, Hodgson TA, Kopstein AN. The economic costs of illness: replication and update. *Health Care Financing Rev* 1985;7:61–80.
16. Rice DP, Mackenzie and Associates. *Cost of injury in the United States: a report to Congress.* San Francisco, CA: Institute for Health & Aging, University of California and Injury Prevention Center, The Johns Hopkins University, 1989.
17. Hodgson TA. Cost of illness in cost-effectiveness analysis: a review of the methodology. *PharmacoEconomics* 1994;6(6):536–52.
18. Guinan ME, Farnhan PG, Holtgrave DR. Estimating the value of preventing a human immunodeficiency virus infection. *Am J Prev Med* 1994;10:1–4.
19. Finkler SA. The distinction between cost and charges. *Ann Intern Med* 1982;96:102–9.
20. U.S. Bureau of the Census. *Statistical abstract of the United States: 1994* (114th ed). Washington, D.C.: 1994.
21. Elixhauser A (ed.) Health care cost-benefit and cost-effectiveness analysis (CBA/ CEA) from 1979 to 1990: a bibliography. *Med Care* 1993;31(7):suppl. JS2– JS150.
22. Landefeld JS, Seskin EP. The economic value of life: linking theory to practice. *Am J Public Health* June 1982;72(6):555–66.
23. Haddix AC, Hillis SD, Kassler WJ. The cost-effectiveness of azithromycin for *Chlamydia trachomatis* infections in women. *J Sexually Transmitted Dis* 1995; 22:174–80.

BIBLIOGRAPHY

Brown K, Burrows C. The sixth stool test: $47 million that never was. *J Health Economics* 1990;9:429–45.
Detsky AS, Nagalie G. A clinician's guide to cost-effectiveness analysis. *Ann Intern Med* 1990;113(2):147–54.
Eisenberg JM. New drugs and clinical economics: analysis of cost-effectiveness in the assessment of pharmaceutical innovations. *Rev Infect Dis* 1984;6(supp4): S905–8.
Health care cost-benefit and cost-effectiveness analysis (CBA/CEA) from 1979 to 1990: a bibliography. *Med Care* 1993;31(7): supplement (July) JS2–JS150.
Kaewsonthi S, Harding A. Cost and performance of malaria surveillance in Thailand. *Social Science Med* 1984;19(10):1081–97.
Lipscomb J. Time preference for health in cost-effectiveness analysis. *Med Care* 1989;27(supp 3):S233–53.
Logan, AG et al. Cost-effectiveness of worksite hypertension treatment program. *Hypertension* 1981;3(2):211–18.
Mooney G, Creese A. Cost and cost-effectiveness analysis of health interventions. *Health Sector Priorities Review* HSPR-23 World Bank, November, 1990.
Neuhauser D, Lewicki AM. What do we gain from the sixth stool guaiac? *N Engl J Med* 1975;293:226–28.

Phelps CE, Mushlin AI. On the (near) equivalence of cost-effectiveness and cost-benefit analyses. *Int J Technology Assessment in Health Care* 1991;7(1):12–21.

Shepard DS et al. Cost-effectiveness of the expanded programme on immunization in the Ivory Coast: a preliminary assessment. *Soc Sci Med* 1986;22(3):369–77.

Sudre P, Breman JG, McFarland DA, Koplan JP. Treatment of chloroquine-resistant malaria in African children: a cost-effectiveness analysis. *Int J Epidemiol* 1992;21(1):146–54.

Udvarhelyi IS, Colditz GA, Rai A, Epstein AM. Cost-effectiveness and cost-benefit analyses in the medical literature; are the methods being used correctly? *Ann Intern Med* 1992;116:238–44.

9

Cost-Utility Analysis

ERIK DASBACH
STEVEN M. TEUTSCH

Cost-utility analysis (CUA) is a specific kind of cost-effectiveness analysis. CUA is appropriate[1] when

- Quality of life is *the* important outcome
- Quality of life is *an* important outcome
- The program being evaluated affects both morbidity and mortality
- The programs being compared have a wide range of different outcomes
- The program being evaluated is being compared with a program that has already been evaluated using CUA

Cost-utility analysis allows comparison across health interventions and has been applied in a diverse array of interventions including postpartum use of anti-D gamma globulin,[2] smoking cessation,[3] and phenylketonuria screening.[4]

This chapter presents:

1. A discussion of why and how quality-adjusted life years (QALYs) are measured
2. Sources of data for measuring QALYs
3. An example of using QALYs in a CUA

The chapter focuses on a specific aspect of cost-effectiveness analysis, namely, quality-of-life adjustments, rather than presenting step-by-step information on performing an analysis as we did for CBA and CEA. Except for the added feature of quality-of-life adjustments, the methods for conducting CUA parallel those for CEA (see chapter 8).

DEFINITION OF COST-UTILITY ANALYSIS AND COMPARISON WITH COST-EFFECTIVENESS ANALYSIS

CUA differs from CEA in the way the health outcomes are measured. In CUA, the results are usually reported as cost per QALY gained. However, in CUA, if the utility measurement includes the value for lost productivity, productivity losses should not be included in the numerator because this will result in double counting. If the utility measurement does not take into account utility lost as the result of a change in productivity due to an illness, productivity losses should be included in the net cost calculation in the numerator.

Recommendation: The numerator in a cost-utility analysis should only include direct medical and nonmedical costs unless the utility measurement in the denominator does not incorporate productivity losses.

Once the quantitative measure of the health outcome has been adjusted for qualitative changes, the CUA is conducted as one would conduct a standard cost-effectiveness analysis.

WHY MEASURE QUALITY OF LIFE?

To compare health programs on the basis of economic value, a standard measure must be used. Sometimes the natural units of measure for different health interventions are similar and programs can be easily compared using CEA. For example, when comparing two interventions designed to reduce neural tube defects, a natural unit of measure might be the number of neural tube defects averted.

For other health interventions, however, natural units of measure may not be similar and a straightforward comparison will therefore not be possible. For example, a program designed to reduce birth defects and a program to reduce lead toxicity among children have very different natural units of outcome measure (e.g., number of birth defects averted compared with IQ levels of children). Although both interventions address the health of children, program results cannot simply be compared. Thus a standard metric must be used to allow comparison. In other cases, interventions may have multiple outcomes, all of which may need to be assessed in a single summary outcome measure.

Suitable measures must address changes in *length* of life as well as in *quality* of life. Several approaches have been developed that include both prognosis and preferences for health states. Among the specific instruments that have been developed for combining quantity and quality of life into a single, summary index are the Quality of Well-Being (QWB) Scale, the Health Utility Index (HUI), and the Years of Healthy Life (YHL). These approaches provide information about health-related quality of life that is expressed in terms of years of healthy life, sometimes also referred to as quality-adjusted life years (QALYs), healthy life years, or disability-adjusted life years (DALYs).

Using QALYs is most appropriate when quality of life is *the* important outcome in a study, e.g., in a program designed to improve social functioning of persons with mental disabilities. Also, when quality of life is *an* important outcome, though not necessarily the only important outcome, a CUA using QALYs can provide useful data, because QALYs can combine multiple outcomes in a single measure.

When a program affects both morbidity and mortality, QALYs can be used to assess the overall program outcomes. For example, an exercise program to reduce the mortality from coronary artery disease may also reduce the incidence. Thus the standardized quality-of-life metrics provide a means for comparing health programs on the basis of cost-effectiveness, considering both quality and length of life.

HOW QALYs ARE MEASURED

Mathematically, QALYs are calculated as the sum of the product of the number of years of life and the quality of life in each of those years. One life year in optimal health is assigned a value of 1. Death is given a value of 0. The value of a year in less than perfect health is given a value between 0 and 1. Thus the number of QALYs is calculated as Number of QALYs = Sum of the years of life in each health state × Quality of life in each health state. For example, in the case of an individual with cancer, CUA would consider not only the absolute number of years of survival after diagnosis but also how much pain and disability an individual suffered during those years. The utility measure for a cancer patient who was bedridden and in extreme pain might be only *0.3*, when quality of life has been taken into consideration.

The QALY formula provides a way to compare health outcomes when both quality and length of life are affected. Measuring duration of life is straightforward. However, measuring the value of the quality of life associated with a particular state of health requires that individuals or groups be studied to determine how a particular state of health is valued by that individual or group. The value assigned to quality of life is referred to as *health utility*.

QALYs provide a method for comparing outcomes that have widely varying results. To illustrate, consider the health outcomes of two different programs to prevent amputations due to diabetes. The baseline program achieves no improvement but delays the time until the patient must have an amputation, whereas a foot-care program provides improved function and no amputation. The quality of life for an individual who must have a limb amputated would be valued very differently from that for a person enrolled in the foot-care program. If only cost measures were used, an amputation program might appear to be a less expensive option than foot-care education over the life of an individual with diabetes. In this example—as in many public health interventions—quality of life is critical in assessing possible outcomes.

QALYs are also useful in integrating results of interventions that have several outcomes. For example, a smoking-cessation program may result in changes in both length of life and quality of life, because of such associated health problems as emphysema, coronary artery disease, and cancer. Assessing the changes in morbidity and mortality from each of these disease conditions individually can be difficult to interpret. Using QALYs allows the overall quality of life to be assessed, rather than limiting assessment to unidimensional changes in health status.

The quality weights for use in calculating QALYs should be based on the relative preferences that individuals have for the various health outcomes. That is, outcomes that are more preferred should have higher weights. Utility theory provides a well-established approach for the measurement of preferences.[5-7] Utilities measured in accord with this theory have interval scale properties, a necessary requirement for the calculation and use of QALYs. For health state utilities, perfect health is assigned a value of 1 and death is assigned a value of 0.

Health state utilities, then, are an expression of health-related quality of life; and QALYs are an expression of health utility and length of life combined. In decision analysis of health outcomes, two approaches have been used to assign health utilities: the direct approach and the indirect approach (see below). Generally, the economic viewpoint of an analysis dictates the appropriate method for measuring health utilities.

THE DIRECT APPROACH TO MEASURING HEALTH UTILITIES

The *direct approach* to health utilities measures how an individual values a given health state. Because of this, the direct approach is most appropriate for clinical decision analysis (i.e., individual decision making). With the direct approach, health utilities are elicited directly from an individual by using a standard technique, such as the "standard gamble," "time trade-off," or "rating-scale."

The *standard gamble* approach is a lottery-based approach. In this technique, shown in Figure 9.1, an individual is asked to choose between a less desirable (but certain) chronic health state (State B_i) and a gamble offering a certain probability of a worse health state (Dead) or having an improved state of health (Healthy).

For example, a patient might be given the choice of undergoing surgery or progressing to a certain chronic health state B_i. With surgery, the possible outcomes are a healthy life with a probability of p or death, with a probability of $1 - p$. To construct the standard gamble model, the patient would be asked, "Would you prefer no surgery if you were certain that this choice would lead to survival for N years with a chronic health condition, or would you prefer to undergo surgery if the chances of surviving Y years with full health were 50% and the chance of death were 50% (a gamble with a 50% chance of the best possible outcome)?" An individual would then choose one of the two treatment options on the basis of the possible outcomes.

Next, the interviewer would continue to ask the same question but would vary the probability of the gamble. If the individual in the above example chose surgery, the interviewer might then ask, "What if your chances of surviving with full health were 25% rather than 50%?" This process would continue until the individual's response indicated indifference to the options of the certain state of health and the gamble. The utility would measure the point at which the person would be neutral between the two choices.

The standard gamble is considered a standard elicitation method because its theoretical foundations are rooted in the axioms of expected utility theory. If an

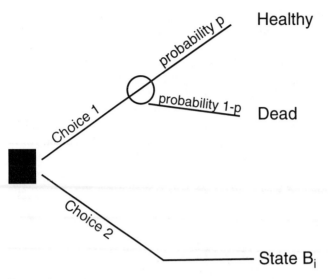

Figure 9.1 Standard gamble for eliciting utilities for a chronic health state (*4*).

individual's responses satisfy the axioms for calculating expected utility, the standard gamble elicitation method results in a measure with interval scale properties.

Time Trade-Off

Because the standard gamble technique may be difficult to administer, the time trade-off technique, which many believe to be easier to administer, was developed.[8] The time trade-off technique is used to determine how many years of life in excellent health are equivalent to life with a less desirable health state. To continue the above example, a patient might be asked to choose between two alternatives: (1) the no surgery option that results in a chronic health condition with a life expectancy of t years, or (2) the surgery option with the chance for full health with a life expectancy of x, where $x \langle t$. Time x is varied until the individual is indifferent between the choice of surgery of no surgery. Figure 9.2

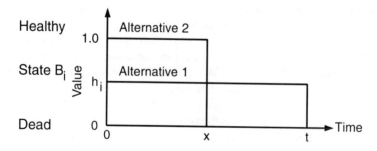

Figure 9.2 Time trade-off for a chronic health condition preferred to death (*4*).

illustrates the case for this example where the time trade-off for a chronic health condition is preferred to death. The preference value h_i for state B_i is $h_i = x/t$.[9] The time trade-off technique differs from the standard gamble in that the individual is presented with a choice that does not involve risk. In the example with the standard gamble, probability was stated as a 50% chance for the best outcome. In the time trade-off example, both outcomes were presented as certain. As a result, the time trade-off technique measures *preference value* and does not, therefore, satisfy the axioms of expected utility theory.

Rating Scale

Another method that has been used to elicit health utilities is the rating-scale technique. Like the time trade-off technique, the rating-scale technique does not involve judgments about risky outcomes. The rating-scale technique is, therefore, also a measure of preference.

In the rating-scale technique, an individual directly relates a health state to a linear scale for example from 0 to 100, where 0 corresponds to the least desirable health state (e.g., death), and 100 corresponds to the most desirable state of health (i.e., excellent health). This kind of scale has been called a *feeling thermometer*.[10] In addition to the feeling thermometer, a card is used to describe a particular state of health. The analyst instructs an individual to place various cards on the scale such that each card's distance from the end points on the feeling thermometer corresponds to her or his feelings about the relative differences in desirability among the levels. The numerical values from the feeling thermometer are then converted to utility values, e.g., values on a scale of 0 to 1. Thus, if the individual places a card at 50, the utility for the health state is 0.5 on a scale of 0 to 1. The individual creates an interval scale using judgments about the desirability of a particular state of health relative to all the other possible states of health.

INDIRECT APPROACH TO MEASURING HEALTH UTILITIES

In contrast to the direct approach, the *indirect approach* measures how the general public, rather than an individual, values a given health state. Because it reflects the values of the general public, the indirect approach is more appropriate for CUAs in public health than the direct approach.

Utilities for the general public as a group may also be estimated using data collection methods that combine different dimensions of health to compute a series of health-utility values. Once the utility values and weights are developed for each dimension, they can then be combined mathematically into a single function known as a *multiattribute-utility (MAU) model*. For example, one model characterized health according to four dimensions: physical function, role function, social-emotional function, and other coexisting health problems.[10] With this model, descriptions were developed for each of the four dimensions for a particular health condition. In one study of multiple sclerosis, for example, physical function was described as "being able to get around the house, yard, neighborhood, or community without help; [needing] mechanical aids to walk or get around."[10] Descriptions were also developed for each of the other three dimensions. After descriptions of the dimensions were developed, utility values were developed for all of the four dimensions.

In constructing a Health Utility Index, one of the direct methods described above can be used to solicit information from individuals. Group-utility values can then be derived by averaging responses from individuals. The value of different aspects of state of health can also be weighted according to their relative contributions to the overall utility of a general health state. Like the utility functions, the weights can be derived by using direct-elicitation techniques with individuals and deriving group weights by averaging individual weights.

Another frequently used MAU model is called the *Quality of Well-Being Index (QWB)*. With an appropriate model, a group-utility index can be constructed for health conditions of interest and used to develop utility values the general public has for a particular disease condition. Group-utility values are expressed in numbers ranging from 0 to 1 so they may be easily inserted into the basic equation for calculating QALYs.

Developing and administering a Health Utility Index is one way to collect data on group-utility values for particular health conditions. Data for measuring utilities and QALYs are available from various sources. Some sources of data, their advantages, and their limitations are discussed below.

SOURCES OF DATA FOR MEASURING QALYs

Collection of Primary Data

To obtain the quality-adjusted health outcomes for the denominator of the CUA it is necessary to measure quality weights for all of the health outcomes or health states in all alternatives in the decision model. Data for measuring QALYs can be obtained through primary data collection. When collecting primary data, one can conduct direct measurement on individuals in the health states of interest. It is necessary to find patients with the various conditions and use a utility measurement instrument (e.g., standard gamble) to measure their utility for their condition.

An alternative is to conduct direct measurements on individuals who have some experience or knowledge of the health states. It is desirable to find patients who have had the disease or condition of interest and have some knowledge about the various health states. Again, a utility measurement instrument (e.g., standard gamble) is used to measure their utility for all the states.

The third alternative is to administer a Health Utility Index to a random sample of the general population. Utilities are measured for the health states of interest as described above.

Primary collection of quality adjustment weights is often not feasible for prevention-effectiveness studies, owing to time and cost constraints. However, a number of instruments are available to facilitate primary data collection. These include the QWB, the HUI, the Rosser, and the EuroQol. The most widely used and tested is the Quality of Well-Being Index (QWB). CDC's Behavioral Risk Factor Surveillance System (BRFSS) has developed a telephone interview version. The drawback of using the QWB or other detailed instruments to collect utility data is that substantial resources are required to train interviewers, interview subjects, and process the data. The QWB would be a more feasible vehicle for collecting data if the instrument were shorter and self-administered. An approach has been developed that uses the short-form health interview survey (SF-36) quality-of-life instrument developed from measures used in the Health Insurance Experiment as a data-collection medium for the QWB.[11,12] The two instruments have been compared, and a translation function developed that maps the SF-36 into the QWB, which assesses the level of disability. The World Bank has used a different measure, the disability-adjusted life year (DALY) as a standard measure for comparing health outcomes for various health conditions.[13,14] DALYs, however, were developed using utilities from an expert panel and lack the rigor of other preference measures.

DATA FROM OTHER SOURCES

Data from National Surveys

If primary data cannot feasibly be obtained, information from national surveys, such as administered by NCHS can be used. NCHS has developed a number of algorithms for mapping the National Health and Nutrition Examination Survey, National Medical Expenditures Survey, and National Health Interview Survey data into the QWB as well as into the Health Utility Index (HUI).[15]

These models of health-related quality of life are based on a retrospective analysis of national survey data and are useful for examining relationships between health-related quality of life and socioeconomic or disease states within the specific surveys.[16] They have also been useful for guiding the development of a measure that can be estimated directly from data collected in the National Health Interview Survey. This measure, called the Years of Healthy Life, was developed in response to the need to monitor changes in the healthy life span as set forth in *Healthy people 2000*.[17] Information from this utility-based measure may be useful for supplying population-based estimates of utilities for different health conditions.[18]

Data from Other Surveys

Another source of utility data is reports of studies of utilities. The drawback with many of these studies is that they are not population-based. A set of tables of health utilities for persons with prevalent health conditions is provided in Table 9.1, for example.[19]

Table 9.1   Age-Adjusted Mean Scores on the QWB for Persons Reporting Being Affected or Not by Various Health Conditons in the Past Year

Condition	n	Means for Persons Affected by the Condition		n	Means for Persons Unaffected by the Condition	
		Mean Score[a]	95% Confidence Interval for the Mean		Mean Score[a]	95% Confidence Interval for the Mean
Arthritis	618	0.679	(0.68,0.70)	738	0.75	(0.75,0.76)
Gout	56	0.74	(0.72,0.77)	1300	0.72	(0.72,0.73)
Severe back pain	249	0.67	(0.66,0.68)	1107	0.74	(0.73,0.74)
Severe neck pain	103	0.68	(0.66,0.69)	1253	0.73	(0.72,0.73)
Migraine	73	0.70	(0.68,0.72)	1283	0.73	(0.72,0.73)
Angina	68	0.66	(0.64,0.69)	1283	0.73	(0.72,0.73)
Congestive heart failure	30	0.63	(0.59,0.67)	1326	0.73	(0.72,0.73)
Myocardial infarction	20	0.64	(0.60,0.68)	1336	0.73	(0.72,0.73)
Stroke	13	0.68	(0.62,0.73)	1343	0.73	(0.72,0.73)
Hypertension	495	0.72	(0.71,0.73)	861	0.73	(0.72,0.74)
Hyperlipidemia	110	0.74	(0.72,0.76)	1246	0.72	(0.72,0.73)
Cataract	327	0.71	(0.70,0.72)	1029	0.73	(0.72,0.74)
Glaucoma	68	0.70	(0.67,0.72)	1288	0.73	(0.72,0.73)
Macular degeneration	44	0.67	(0.64,0.70)	1312	0.73	(0.72,0.73)
Diabetes (insulin)	36	0.66	(0.63,0.69)	1320	0.73	(0.72,0.73)
Diabetes (noninsulin)	88	0.70	(0.68,0.72)	1268	0.73	(0.72,0.73)
Asthma	46	0.68	(0.65,0.71)	1310	0.73	(0.72,0.73)
Emphysema	40	0.67	(0.63,0.70)	1315	0.73	(0.72,0.73)
Chronic bronchitis	46	0.67	(0.65,0.70)	1309	0.73	(0.72,0.73)
Chronic sinusitis	95	0.72	(0.70,0.74)	1261	0.73	(0.72,0.73)
Depression	62	0.65	(0.63,0.68)	1294	0.73	(0.72,0.73)
Anxiety	54	0.68	(0.65,0.70)	1302	0.73	(0.72,0.73)
Ulcer	77	0.67	(0.65,0.69)	1279	0.73	(0.72,0.73)
Colitis	51	0.70	(0.67,0.73)	1305	0.73	(0.72,0.73)
Hiatal hernia	46	0.70	(0.67,0.72)	1310	0.73	(0.72,0.73)
Sleep disorder	136	0.68	(0.66,0.69)	1220	0.73	(0.73,0.74)
Thyroid disorder	88	0.70	(0.68,0.72)	1268	0.73	(0.72,0.73)
Miscellaneous allergies	280	0.72	(0.69,0.76)	1328	0.73	(0.72,0.73)

[a] All means adjusted to 64.0 years, the overall sample mean age; best = 1.0; worst = 0.0. Confidence intervals computed using Regress command in MINITAB Vax/VMS version 7.1, (c)1989 Minitab, Inc.
Source: Fryback et al. Medical Decision Making 13(2).

CONDUCTING A COST-UTILITY ANALYSIS

In the sections below, a simplified, hypothetical example of a CUA to evaluate a health program designed to prevent chronic disease at birth is presented. Assuming that the primary difference between a CEA and a CUA is the measure used to evaluate effectiveness, this example focuses only on how QALYs are measured and used in a CUA.

The first step is to identify the options being evaluated. In this example, there are two options. Option A is a program that prevents chronic disease (X) at birth. Option B is a no-program option that would result in the natural progression of chronic disease (X) over an expected lifetime with the disease. The second step is to identify the health states that Option A and Option B will follow. A minimum set of health states should include all those that result in a change in quality of life or a change in expenditure of resources. In this example, two health states are assumed: excellent health and chronic disease X.

Next, life expectancy should be estimated. In this example, two assumptions are made: (1) the life expectancy of an individual for whom chronic disease X has been prevented is 75 years (Option A), and (2) the life expectancy of an individual with chronic disease X from birth is 30 years (Option B).

The utility of living in excellent health is 1.0. In this example, it is assumed that the utility associated with living with chronic disease X (Option B) is similar to living with noninsulin-dependent diabetes. Thus the corresponding utility found in Table 9.1 (i.e., 0.70) is used for the calculations.

Figure 9.3 depicts the results of the calculations used to determine the incremental gain in QALYs when Option A is chosen instead of Option B. Option A accrues 75 QALYs (75 years × 1 QALY/yr). Option B, in contrast, accrues 21 QALYs (30 years × 0.70 QALY/yr). Thus, Option A gains 54 QALYs over Option B. This substantial gain would decrease if discounting were incorporated.

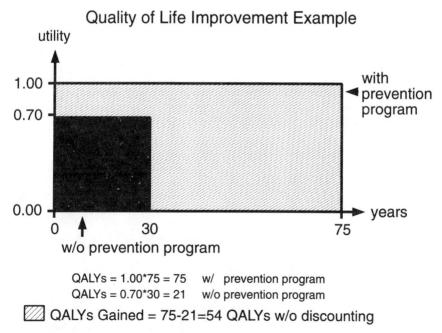

Figure 9.3 Measuring effectiveness with QALYs.

CONCLUSION

CUA is similar to other methods of economic analysis because it examines the number of health outcomes. It also includes measures of the length of life and quality of life, rather than just the number of individuals affected by a program. Because length of life is a factor, CUA tends to favor interventions aimed at conditions affecting younger persons. It differs from CEA and CBA by including measures of the quality of life. Measuring quality of life is both complex and difficult. The methods presented in this chapter convey some options for consideration, but better techniques are needed. Agreement on standardized methods for collecting, applying, and interpreting quality-of-life data may also make CUA more useful for analysts and decision makers. Adding quality of life to an economic analysis adds another layer of analytic complexity and requires interpretation that may be confusing for persons unfamiliar with CUA methods.

CUA does, however, provide a method for comparing different health interventions in a way that considers both quality of life and length of life. CUA can provide useful information in the overall process of decision making and policy development. As with each method described in this book, economic analysis and decision analysis do not make decisions. They simply provide information to help decision makers clarify issues, compare options, and evaluate options. Public health decisions require a holistic approach to decision making that includes not only cost information, but consideration of ethical, legal, and distributional issues as well.

REFERENCES

1. Drummond MF, Stoddard GL, Torrance GW. *Methods for the economic evaluation of health care programmes.* Oxford: Oxford University Press, 1987.
2. Torrance GW, Zipursky A. Cost effectiveness analysis of treatment with anti-D. Cost effectiveness of antepartum prevention of Rh immunization. *Clin Perinatol* 1984, 11(2): 267–81.
3. Williams A. The importance of quality of life in policy decisions. in *Quality of Life: Assessment and Application.* Walker SR, Rosser RM (eds). Lancaster, England: MTP Press, 279–90, 1988.
4. Bush JW, Chen MM, Patrick DL. Health status index in cost-effectiveness: analysis of PKU program in *Health Status Indexes.* Berg R (eds). Chicago: Hospital Research and Educational Trust, 172–208, 1973.
5. von Neumann J, Morgenstern O. *Theory of games and economic behavior.* New York: John Wiley and Sons, 1944.
6. Torrance GW. Measurement of health state utilities for economic appraisal: a review. *J Health Economics* 1986;5:1–30.
7. Torrance GW, Feeny DH. Utilities and quality-adjusted life years. *Int J Technology Assessment in Health Care* 1989;5:559–75.
8. Torrance GW, Thomas WH, Sackett DL. A utility maximization model for evaluation of health care programs. *Health Services Res* 1972;7(2):118–33.

9. Torrance GW. Measurement of health state utilities for economic appraisal: a review. *J Health Economics* 1986;5:1–30.
10. Torrance GW, Boyle MH, Horwood SP. Application of multi-attribute utility theory to measure social preferences for health states. *Operations Res* 1982;30(6):1043–69.
11. Fryback DG, Dasbach E, Klein BEK, Martin PA, Dorn N, Peterson K. *Health assessment by SF-36, quality of well-being index, and time tradeoffs: predicting one measure from another.* Presentation at fourteenth annual meeting of the Society for Medical Decision Making, 1992.
12. Ware JE Jr, Sherbourne CD. The MOS 36-item short-form health survey (SF-36): conceptual framework and item selection. *Med Care* 1992;30(6):473–83.
13. World Bank. *World development report 1993.* New York: Oxford University Press, 1993.
14. Murray CJL. Quantifying the burden of disease: the technical basis for disability-adjusted life years. *Bull WHO* 1994 77:429–45.
15. Erickson P, Kendall EA, Anderson JP, Kaplan RM. Using composite health status measures to assess the nation's health. *Med Care* 1987; 27 (Suppl 3):S66–S77.
16. Erickson P, Kendall EA, Odle MP, Torrance GW. *Assessing health-related quality of life in the National Health and Nutrition Examination Survey.* National Center for Health Statistics, Hyattsville, MD, 1992.
17. Erickson P, Wilson R, Shannon I. Years of healthy life. *Statistical Note Number 7.* National Center for Health Statistics, Hyattsville, MD, 1995.
18. Public Health Service. *Healthy people 2000: national health promotion and disease prevention objectives—full report with commentary.* Washington, D.C.: U.S. Department of Health and Human Services, Public Health Service; DHHS publication no. (PHS)91-50212, 1991.
19. Fryback DG, Dasbach E, Klein R, Klein BE, Dorn N, Peterson K. The Beaver Dam Health Outcomes Study: initial catalog of health-state quality factors. *Med Decision Making* 1993;13(2):89–102.

BIBLIOGRAPHY

Boyle MH et al. Economic evaluation of neonatal intensive care of very-low-birth-weight infants. *N Engl J Med* 1983;308:1330–37.
Carr-Hill R. Background material for the workshop on QALYs: assumptions of the QALY procedure. *Soc Sci Med* 1989;29(3):469–77.
Donaldson C et al. Should QALYs be programme-specific? *J Health Economics* 1988;7:239–57.
Drummond MF. Resource allocation decisions in health care: a role for quality of life assessments? *J Chronic Dis* 1987;40(6)605–19.
Feeny DH, Torrance GW. Incorporating utility-based quality-of-life assessment measures in clinical trials. *Med Care* 1989; 27(3) Suppl S190–204.
Harris J. Life: quality, value and justice. *Health Policy* 1988;10(3):259–66.
Harris J. QALYfying the value of life. *J Med Ethics* 1987;13(3):117–23.
Kaplan RM, Bush JW, Berry CC. Health status: types of validity and the index of well-being. *Health Services Res,* 1976.
La Puma J, Lawlor EF. Quality-adjusted life-years ethical implications for physicians and policymakers. *JAMA* 1990;263(21):2917–21.

Loomes G, McKenzie L. The use of QALYs in health care decision making. *Soc Sci Med* 1989;28(4):299–308.

Mehrez A, Gafni A. Quality-adjusted life years, utility theory, and healthy-year equivalents. *Med Decision Making* 1989;9(2):142–49.

Mehrez A, Gafni A. Quality-adjusted life years, utility theory, and healthy-year equivalents. *Med Decision Making* 1990;10(2):148–49 (Erratum).

Miyamoto JM, Eraker SA. Parameter estimates for a QALY utility model. *Med Decision Making* 1985;5(2):191–213.

Nord E. Methods of quality adjustment of life years. *Soc Sci Med* 1992; 34(5):559–69.

Pliskin J, Shepard D, Weinstein M. Utility functions for life years and health status. *Operations Research* 1980;28:206–24.

Quirk JP. *Intermediate microeconomics.* Chicago: Science Research Associates, 1983.

Sackett DL, Torrance GW. The utility of different health states as perceived by the general public. *J Chronic Dis* 1978;31:697–704.

Stewart AL, Ware JE Jr (eds). *Measuring functioning and well-being: the medical outcomes study approach.* Durham, NC: Duke University Press, 1992.

Torrance GW. Measurement of health state utilities for economic appraisal: a review. *J Health Economics* 1986;5:1–30.

Torrance GW, Boyle MH, Horwood SP. Application of multi-attribute utility theory to measure social preferences for health states. *Operations Research* 1982; 30(6):1043–69.

Torrance GW, Feeny DH. Utilities and quality-adjusted life years. *Int J Technology Assessment in Health Care* 1989;5(4):559–75.

Wagstaff A. QALYs and the equity-efficiency trade-off. *J Health Economics* 1991;10:21–41.

Walker SR, Rosser RM. *Quality of life: assessment and application.* Lancaster, PA: MTP Press, 1988.

APPENDIX A
Glossary

adequacy When applied to an intervention, the ratio of the expected number of potentially preventable cases to the number of cases that would occur in the absence of an intervention.

adverse event (outcome) Premature death or morbidity.

analytic hierarchy approach A decision-aiding approach in which the attributes of an outcome are ranked in order of importance.

analytic horizon The time period over which the costs and benefits of health outcomes that occur as a result of the intervention are considered.

annuitizing Determining a constant annual value of a capital item for the life of the capital investment.

attributable risk The theoretical reduction in the rate or number of cases of an adverse outcome that can be achieved by elimination of a risk factor.

audience The consumer of the study results. Defined as policy decision makers, program decision makers, or others such as patients, health-care workers, media, other researchers, and the general public.

average cost See **cost.**

average cost-effectiveness See **cost-effectiveness analysis.**

averaging-out-and-folding-back In decision analysis, a series of mathematical computations of probability values multiplied by utility estimates and summed to average out the expected value of the branches leading out of each chance node. The results are then folded back from right to left until a value is found for each decision option.

baseline comparator One of the alternative prevention strategies in a decision analysis. May be either the existing-program/strategy alternative or a no-program/strategy alternative, if no program exists at the time of the intervention.

behavioral prevention strategies Strategies that require that an individual make a personal effort to change life-style, such as exercise and dietary improvements.

benefit-cost ratio   A mathematical comparison of the benefits divided by the costs of a project or intervention. When the benefit-cost ratio is greater than 1, benefits exceed costs.

best- and worst-case scenario   A type of sensitivity analysis where the decision tree model can be used to calculate low- or high-range values that favor one option and recalculated using values that favor another option.

capital costs   The cost of assets with a productive life of more than 1 year required by a program (e.g., equipment, buildings, and land).

chance node   In a decision tree, an event which occurs as a consequence of the decision but over which one has no control. Usually drawn as a circle.

clinical prevention strategies   Interventions conveyed by a health-care provider to a patient, often within a clinical setting, such as vaccinations, screening and treatment for diabetic eye disease, and monitoring of tuberculosis treatment.

cohort   Any defined group of persons selected for a special purpose or study.

consumer market studies   The determination of the value of nonmarket resources from reference to similar commodities for which a market exists in the context of estimating willingness-to-pay (WTP) values of health outcomes.

consumer price index (CPI)   Measures relative changes over time in the prices of a specified set of goods and services purchased by households on a regular basis.

contingent valuation studies   The use of surveys of individuals conducted in the context of a hypothetical market situation to elicit consumer valuation of goods and services. Used to estimate the willingness-to-pay (WTP) values of health outcomes.

cost   A measure of what must be given up to acquire or produce something. Economic costs can be differentiated in the following manner:

> **total cost (TC)**   Sum of the costs of producing a particular quantity of output.

> **fixed cost (FC)**   Costs which do not vary with the quantity of output in the short run, e.g., rent, utilities, and administrative salaries.

> **variable cost (VC)**   Costs which vary with the level of output and which responds proportionately to change in volume of activity.

> **average cost (AC)**   The total cost divided by the total output. Reported as the cost per unit of output.

> **marginal cost (MC)**   The additional cost of an intervention to produce one additional unit of output. An intraprogram measure.

> **incremental cost (IC)**   When interventions are ranked in ascending order of effectiveness, the additional cost to the next most effective

intervention of producing another unit of output. An interprogram measure.

incidence-based   See **incidence-based cost.**

prevalence-based   See **prevalence-based cost.**

cost analysis   The process of estimating the cost of prevention activities, also called **cost identification.**

cost-benefit analysis (CBA)   A type of economic analysis in which all costs and benefits are converted into monetary (dollar) values and results are expressed as either the net present value or the dollars of benefits per dollars expended.

cost-effectiveness analysis (CEA)   An economic analysis in which all costs are related to a single, common effect. Results are usually stated as additional cost expended per additional health outcome achieved. Results can be categorized in one of or all of the following ways:

> **average cost-effectiveness**   The total cost of an intervention divided by the health outcomes produced by that intervention.

> **marginal cost-effectiveness**   The additional cost incurred by an intervention to produce an additional unit of the health outcome.

> **incremental cost-effectiveness**   When strategies are ranked in order of effectiveness, the additional cost incurred by the next most effective strategy to produce an additional unit of the health outcome.

cost identification   See **cost analysis.**

cost-of-illness (COI) methodology   An approach to estimate the costs of a health intervention in which two types of costs are collected: the direct medical and nonmedical costs associated with the illness and the indirect costs associated with lost productivity due to morbidity or premature mortality.

cost-utility analysis (CUA)   A type of cost-effectiveness analysis in which benefits are expressed as the number of life years saved adjusted to account for loss of quality from morbidity of the health outcome or side effects from the intervention. The most common measure in CUA is the **quality-adjusted life year (QALY).**

decision analysis   An explicit, quantitative, systematic approach to decision making under conditions of uncertainty.

decision node   In a decision tree, the first point of choice, usually drawn as a box.

decision tree models   A graphic representation of how possible choices in a decision analysis relate (stochastically) to the possible outcomes.

delphi process   An iterative consensus process used to determine the "best estimate" of professionals in the field. This process is often used in decision analysis to estimate the probability that an event will occur or the valuation of costs and benefits of outcomes when there is insufficient data in the published literature.

demonstration settings   A population- or clinic-based environment in which prevention strategies are field tested.

direct costs   The measure of the resources expended for prevention activities or healthcare (compare with **indirect cost**).

> **direct medical costs**   The measure of the resources for medical treatment (e.g., the cost of a physician visit).

> **direct nonmedical costs**   Those costs incurred in connection with a health intervention or illness, but which are not expended for medical care itself (e.g., the transportation costs associated with a physician visit).

discounting   A method for adjusting the value of future costs and benefits to an equivalent value today to account for time preference and opportunity cost, i.e., a dollar today is worth more than a dollar a year from now (even if inflation is not considered).

discount rate   The rate at which future costs and benefits are discounted to account for time preference. See **social discount rate** or **real discount rate**.

distributional effects   The manner in which the costs and benefits of a preventive strategy affect different groups of people in terms of demographics, geographic location, and other descriptive factors.

double counting   When a cost or benefit is captured in more than one measure.

effectiveness   The improvement in health outcome that a prevention strategy can produce in typical community-based settings.

efficacy   The improvement in health outcome that a prevention strategy can produce in expert hands under ideal circumstances.

efficiency   A measure of the relationship between inputs and outputs in a prevention strategy. Efficiency goes beyond effectiveness of a prevention strategy by attempting to identify the maximum health output achievable for a set amount of resources.

etiologic fraction   The proportion of cases in the exposed group presumably attributable to the exposure, appropriate only if the exposed group has a higher risk of disease then the unexposed group.

excess fraction   The fractional excess caseload produced by an exposure.

expected utility   The sum of the products of the preference ranking, i.e., utility for an outcome and the probability that the outcome will occur for all the possible outcomes of a prevention strategy.

expected utility theory   The dominant theory of individual behavior under conditions of uncertainty based on the assumption that, given different alternatives, the alternative with the outcome that has the highest expected utility should be chosen.

expected value The sum of the products of the value of outcomes and the probability of the outcome occurring for all possible outcomes of a prevention strategy.

false negative A person with a condition who tests negative for that condition. See **sensitivity (test).**

false positive A person without a condition who tests positive for that condition. See **specificity (test).**

fixed cost (FC) See **cost.**

health promotion Disease and injury prevention strategies that depend on behavioral change in individuals.

health-related event (HRE) Adverse health condition.

health utility The measure assigned to quality of life.

health utility index A multifaceted measure of utility in which different utility functions (e.g., physical function, role function, social-emotional function, and other coexisting health problems) are weighted and combined to determine an overall preference for a particular outcome.

heuristics Psychological short-cuts in thinking used to simplify complex decisions.

human capital (HC) approach A method for estimating the economic impact of disease, which includes the resources used for medical care and the forgone earnings due to morbidity or premature mortality.

incidence-based cost The total lifetime cost of new cases of a disease or injury that occur during a certain period of time.

incidence rate A measure of the frequency of new cases of disease in a particular population, which occurred during a specified period of time.

incremental analysis A type of comparative analysis used to examine the relationship between the differences in costs and benefits (whether measured in monetary, natural, or quality-adjusted units) between two or more prevention strategies.

incremental cost The additional cost of producing one more additional unit of output by an alternative intervention.

incremental cost-effectiveness See **cost-effectiveness.**

indirect cost The resources forgone either to participate in an intervention or as the result of a health condition (e.g., earnings forgone because of loss of time from work).

inflation   A sustained rise in the general price level.

intangible cost   Cost, such as pain and suffering, for which assigning a monetary value is difficult.

intermediate measure   The measure most directly associated with the intervention being evaluated, generally reported in terms of the service delivered, e.g., patients tested, number of condoms distributed.

league tables   Tables used to rank cost-effectiveness and cost-benefit results for various health conditions, usually in ascending order of cost per unit of outcome.

marginal analysis   A type of analysis that examines the additional cost required to produce an additional unit of output by a prevention strategy.

marginal cost   See **cost.**

marginal cost-effectiveness   See **cost-effectiveness.**

meta-analysis   A systematic, quantitative method for combining information from multiple studies in order to derive the most meaningful answer to a specific question.

Monte Carlo simulation   A type of sensitivity analysis which compares the measure of the central tendency and the variance of results generated by repeated decision tree simulations with the expected values of the probabilities and outcome values for the model.

> **first order**   Runs a cohort through the model with the computer making selections randomly at each chance node based on a single value for the probability. A distribution of the accumulated results provides a measure of the central tendency and the variance.

> **second order**   Runs a cohort through the model a number of times, with the computer making random selections from values in a designated distribution for the probability at the chance node. A distribution of the accumulated results provides a measure of the central tendency and the variance.

multiattribute utility (MAU) model   In a cost-utility analysis (CUA), the mathematical combining of the utility functions and weights for each dimension into one single function.

net present value (NPV)   The sum that results when the discounted value of the costs of a prevention strategy are deducted from the discounted value of the benefits of the strategy.

normative decision-making models   Models in decision making that provide rules by which decisions "should be" made.

opportunity cost   The value of the resources used in providing a specific set of health-care services valued in terms of forgone alternative uses.

outcome measure   The final health consequence, e.g., cases prevented, quality-adjusted life years, of an intervention.

participant cost   Direct and indirect costs borne by the participant in the intervention program. Includes travel and day care expenses, the purchase of intervention units not accounted for in program costs, and forgone wages due to lost time from work.

payer   An individual or organization responsible for payment of health-care costs.

penetrance   The proportion of subjects who might benefit who are reached by the intervention.

perspective   See **societal perspective.**

policy decision makers   Elected officials, agency heads, state and local public health officials, and others responsible for setting public health policy.

population attributable risk   The incidence of a disease or condition in a population that is associated with exposure to the risk factor.

premature mortality   (1) Any preventable death; (2) Deaths that occur before a specified age, most often age 65, or the average life expectancy of a certain population.

prescriptive decision-making models   Models used to guide decision making.

prevalence-based cost   The cost associated with the existing cases of disease or injury that occur during a specified time period.

prevalence   The number of instances of a given disease or condition in a given population at a designated time.

preventable fraction   The proportion of an adverse health outcome that potentially can be eliminated as a result of a prevention strategy.

prevented fraction   The proportion of an adverse health outcome that has been eliminated as a result of a prevention strategy.

prevention   The promotion and preservation of health, the restoration of health when it is impaired, and the minimization of suffering and distress.

>   **primary prevention**   An intervention to reduce risk or exposure to prevent occurence of disease or injury.

>   **secondary prevention**   An intervention to detect and treat a disease before it becomes clinically apparent.

>   **tertiary prevention**   An intervention implemented after a disease or injury is established to prevent sequelae or to minimize suffering.

prevention effectiveness   The systematic assessment of the impact of public health policies, programs, and practices on costs and health outcomes.

preventive medical services   Clinical services provided to patients to reduce or prevent disease, injury, or disability. These are preventive measures provided by a health-care professional to a patient.

preventive strategies (clinical, behavioral, environmental)   A framework for categorizing programs based on how the prevention technology is delivered, i.e., provider to patient (clinical), individual responsibility (behavioral), or alteration in an individual's surroundings (environmental).

primary prevention   See **prevention.**

process measures   The set of criteria used to evaluate an intervention based on the measurement of either the quantity of inputs used, e.g., number of brochures distributed, or the products produced, eg., patients tested, by the intervention.

productivity loss   The value of output not produced due to morbidity or premature mortality.

program decision makers   Users of the results of prevention-effectiveness studies who are responsible for decisions about prevention programs.

program evaluation   An assessment of the processes, impacts, and outcomes of intervention programs, with particular attention paid to the purposes and expectations of stakeholders of the program.

quality-adjusted life years (QALY)   A frequently used outcome measure in cost utility analysis that incorporates the quality or desirability of a health state with the duration of survival. The quality of life is integrated with the length of life by using a multiplicative formula.

quality of well-being (QWB)   A health utility index widely used for cost utility analysis.

rank and scale   A method of valuing utilities whereby outcomes are ranked in order of best to worst and then are assigned numerical values.

rating scale   A method of valuing utilities based on strength of preference.

ratio   A measure of the frequency of one group of events relative to the frequency of a different group of events.

real discount rate   A discount rate that is free from the effects of inflation.

recipients of services (beneficiaries)   Any individual or group who benefits from a prevention strategy; used most often in the context of medical services.

relative risk   The ratio of the incidence rate for a person exposed to a factor to the incidence rate for those not exposed.

required compensation approach   An analytic method that attempts to value the reduction in the risk of a job-related injury by examining the difference in wages for persons in risky occupations versus persons in other occupations.

resource An input in a prevention intervention without which the intervention would not exist or an input in the treatment of a health outcome.

risk The likelihood that a person having specified characteristics (e.g., high blood cholesterol, failure to wear seat belts) will acquire a specified disease or injury.

risk ratio The ratio of the risk among persons with specific risk factors compared to the risk among persons without the risk factors.

safety An assessment of the level and acceptability of risk of adverse outcomes that occur as a result of a prevention technique in the context of a specific prevention strategy and disease or injury outcome.

scrap value The resale value of a capital asset at the end of its useful life.

secondary prevention See **prevention.**

sensitivity (test) The ability of a test to correctly identify those who have the disease. A sensitive test creates few false negatives.

sensitivity analysis Mathematical calculations that isolate factors involved in a decision analysis or economic analysis to indicate the degree of influence each factor has on the outcome of the entire analysis.

> **one-way sensitivity analysis** When only one value is changed.

> **multiway sensitivity analysis** When several values are changed simultaneously.

sequela An abnormal condition resulting from a disease.

shadow price An imputed valuation of a commodity or service for which no market price exists. The social opportunity cost of an outcome.

social discount rate The rate at which society as a whole is willing to trade present costs in exchange for future benefits. Used in prevention-effectiveness studies that take the societal perspective, the lower rate indicates that future benefits are also valued highly in the present (see **discount rate**).

societal perspective The perspective of society as a whole. Economic analyses which take a societal perspective include all benefits of a program regardless of who receives them and all costs regardless of who pays them.

specificity (test) The ability of a test to identify correctly those who do not have the disease. A specific test creates few false positives.

stakeholder An individual or organization with an interest in an intervention or outcome.

standard gamble In cost utility analysis, a lottery-based approach to determining the utility of a particular outcome.

target audience See **audience.**

technology   Techniques, devices, drugs, or procedures used to reduce the risk of an adverse health outcome.

terminal node   In a decision tree, the end point of each sequence of events representing a health outcome. Usually represented by a rectangle.

tertiary prevention   See **prevention.**

threshold analysis   A type of sensitivity analysis that identifies the conditions (e.g., the values of variables) that would have to exist for the expected value or expected utility of two interventions to be equivalent. Threshold analysis is often used to identify the "switch points" at which cost savings begin or end and to indicate the point at which a different decision should be made.

time frame   The specified period in which the intervention strategies are actually applied.

time trade-off   A method of eliciting utilities from an individual perspective based on the willingness to trade time for health.

total cost (TC)   See **cost.**

unnecessary morbidity   Any preventable disease, injury, or disability.

utility   In decision analysis, a quantitative measure of the strength of a preferred outcome.

variable cost (VC)   See **cost.**

wage risk studies   See **required compensation approach.**

welfare economics   The normative aspect of economics. Viewed as an investigation of methods of obtaining an ordering of alternative possible resource allocations. Within the context of prevention effectiveness, it provides the framework for the ranking of prevention strategies by order of net costs and benefits.

willingness-to-pay (WTP)   A method of measuring the value an individual places on reducing risk of death and illness by estimating the maximum dollar amount an individual would pay in a given risk-reducing situation.

REFERENCES

Some definitions adapted from:

Drummond MF, Stoddart GL, Torrance GW. *Methods for the economic evaluation of health care programmes.* Oxford: Oxford University Press, 1987.
Last JM. *A dictionary of epidemiology,* 2nd ed. New York: Oxford University Press, 1988.
Mausner J, Kramer S. *Epidemiology: an introductory text.* Philadelphia: W.B. Saunders Co., 1985.

Pearce DW (ed). *The MIT dictionary of modern economics,* 4th ed. Cambridge: MIT Press, 1994.

Petitti DB. *Meta-analysis, decision analysis, and cost-effectiveness analysis: methods for quantitative synthesis in medicine.* New York: Oxford University Press, 1994.

Principles of epidemiology: Self-study course 3030-G. U.S. DHHS, CDC.

Warner KE, Luce BR. *Cost-benefit and cost-effectiveness analysis in health care: principles, practice, and potential.* Ann Arbor: Health Administration Press, 1982.

APPENDIX B
Software

SMLTREE, by James P. Hollenberg, MD, Cornell University, 1987; 16B Pine Drive North, Roslyn, NY 11576; telephone (212) 746-2873.

Description: This software enables users to construct and analyze complex decision trees and Markov processes. Provides immediate graphic display of all changes in decision trees. Decision trees can be edited after they are constructed.

Although the software is not especially user-friendly, an excellent tutorial is available with the software.

User Manual: 75 pages. Tutorial is provided through an on-screen program. An additional tutorial has been developed by Joanna Siegel (Harvard): Siegel JE, Keaney KM. Introduction to SMLTREE. *Med Decision Making* 1993;13(1): 74–84.

Features: Folding back a tree, Cost-effectiveness (DUAL utility scales), threshold analyses, 2- and 3-way sensitivity analyses, risk analyses, Monte Carlo analyses, and Markov processes.

DATA 2.6, by TreeÅge, 1994; P.O. Box 329, Boston, MA 02199; telephone (617)536-2128.

Description: DATA is an advanced program for generating decision trees. It is user-friendly and provides superior graphics. Versions are available for Windows, DOS, and Macintosh systems. The 2.6 version features sophisticated cost-effectiveness analyses geared toward medical decision making.

User Manual: 181 pages. Tutorial is provided through an on-screen program. Manual is set up to correspond with the tutorial.

Features: Folding back a tree, cost-effectiveness (DUAL utility scale), threshold analyses, 2- and 3-way sensitivity analyses, and Markov processes.

DECISION MAKER, by Stephen G. Pauker, MD, Division of Clinical Decision Making, New England Medical Center, Boston, MA 02111; telephone (617) 350-8402

Description: The program is not intended as a means of learning decision analysis, but is quite user-friendly for those with a basic understanding of decision analysis. The program provides graphic displays of decision trees on the screen. The graphic image can be "navigated," that is, the user can highlight different portions of the tree and evaluate the tree from any vantage point. The capability for manipulation of tree structure allows the analyst to assess quickly the impact of variations in tree structure without having to rebuild a model completely each time it is varied.

User Manual: 82 pages.

Features: Foldback (baseline evaluation), 1-way, 2-way, and 3-way sensitivity analyses, threshold analyses, cost-effectiveness analysis, risk profiles, and Markov simulations.

DECAID, by Gordon F. Pitz, Department of Psychology, Southern Illinois University at Carbondale, Carbondale, IL 62901.

Description: This software is very easy to learn and use. It has been used with beginning classes as a teaching tool for decision analysis concepts. The software is somewhat qualitative in its approach to decision making, e.g., the cursor is used to adjust relative lengths of arrows on the computer screen to indicate probabilities and utilities for possible outcomes rather than having to insert actual numerical values. To structure a decision analysis, the user describes problems and lists concerns or goals. Each concern or attribute uses anchor points for the worst and best outcomes. The program leads the user through a series of judgments reflecting the decision maker's preferences. Importance judgments are also determined. A summary evaluation of the options is then displayed with the expected multiattribute utility for each option.

User Manual: None. Installation instructions and a 3-page outline of the program are included.

FAST*PRO, by David M. Eddy, MD, and Vic Hasselblad, MD, both of the Center for Health Policy Research and Education, Duke University, Durham, NC.

Description: Based on the Confidence Profile Method for meta-analysis, Fast*Pro is intended to estimate parameters important for decisions, such as the outcomes of diseases and the effects of treatments. The role of the software is to help the user synthesize any existing evidence to derive estimates of the parameters the user wants to use in models and decision analysis. The results can be presented as single best estimates or as probability distributions. Developed by health-policy-research experts, the software is geared toward decision making in the health area.

User Manual: 196 pages with some examples.

SUPER-OPTIMIZING POLICY ANALYSIS, by Stewart Nagel and Joyce Nagel, University of Illinois, Political Science Department, 361 Lincoln Hall, 702 S. Wright Street, Urbana, IL. 61801

Description: The software was developed and used for public policy analysis in areas such as minimum-wage subsidies, bicycle-safety-feature requirements, and food-price analysis in China. The intended users include lawyers and judges, and many examples of dispute resolution and negotiated outcomes are provided in the user manual.

The "Super-Optimizing Solution" analysis program concentrates on only four basic options (defined as conservative, liberal, neutral, and super-optimizing). Two basic goals are defined by the user for each option. A 1-to-5-point scale allows the user to rate how conducive each option is to each goal. The program then presents the best conservative option and the best liberal option. Finally, the program finds the solution with the highest total score by applying both conservative and liberal weights.

This solution, the "super-optimizing solution," is intended to present an option that goes beyond compromise, and even beyond a "win/win" situation, illuminating a solution that actually exceeds the expectations of both conservatives and liberals.

User Manual: 85 pages including background information and examples.

CRYSTAL BALL FOR WINDOWS, by Decisioneering, Inc.,1380 Lawrence Street, Suite 520, Denver, CO 80204-9849; telephone (303) 292-2291.

Description: This software is specifically designed for the decision maker who wants to forecast an entire range of results possible for a given situation and perform a risk analysis for each result. Designed more for a quantitative analysis, this program relies heavily on statistical methods and requires the use and knowledge of Microsoft Excel (Lotus 1-2-3 can be used as a substitute). Although familiarity with statistics is helpful, the manual and tutorials provide easy-to-understand descriptions of these concepts. Crystal Ball is helpful only if there are concrete numbers to back up assumptions; qualitative assessments play no role in its calculations.

User Manual: 168 pages.

Features: Monte Carlo simulation, trend charts, and sensitivity charts.

CONTINUOUS RISK, by Nevada Simulations, P.O. Box 32272, Phoenix, AZ 85064-2272.

Description: This software uses a probabilistic programming language for risk and decision analyses. Decision trees allow for 4-parameter probability distributions. Although not specifically targeted for public health decision makers, the software may be appropriate for medical decision analysts who model survival distributions or Markov processes. Runs on DOS and Windows.

EXPERT CHOICE 8.0, by The Decision Support Software Company, 4922 Ellsworth Avenue, Pittsburgh, PA 15213.

Description: This software models complex decisions by organizing the elements of the decision into a hierarchy, through the mathematical theory known as the Analytic Hierarchy Process (AHP). The AHP allows the user to include both quantitative and qualitative data into the decision-making process. The software guides the user in judging the relative importance of criteria, and the preferences for the alternatives defined.

APPENDIX C
HIV Needle-Stick Case Study

The following is a brief synopsis of a case study devised by Sankey Williams of the University of Pennsylvania.

In this case study, you, as the health-care worker, have sustained a needle-stick injury while obtaining blood from an individual who is known to be HIV seropositive. The problem is what to do next. This problem appears to be an appropriate one for applying decision analysis techniques since (a) the choice is not intuitively clear (i.e., it involves complex issues, and information about the relative benefits and risks of the options is uncertain), (b) two or more real and mutually exclusive decision alternatives exist, and (c) the decision is very important for your future health.

The first questions posed by Williams are these: "What are your options?" and "What is known about the consequences of each option?" One option is to do nothing, i.e., wait and see whether you develop HIV antibodies. Another option is to start treatment with one or more antiretroviral agents. If you choose the first option, you must wait at least 6 months before obtaining information that may allow you to be fairly confident that you have not been infected. In the meantime, you must take precautions to prevent your transmitting HIV to others, and you must deal with the anxiety associated with the possibility that you will develop HIV infection because you have not done anything to prevent it since incurring the needle-stick injury.

If you choose the second option and begin treatment with an antiretroviral agent, you still must take precautions and worry, and, in addition, you must accept the inconvenience and potential adverse effects of taking the medication. If you choose treatment, most experts advise taking zidovudine (AZT) 200 mg. every 4 hours for 6 weeks, although other drugs and drug combinations can be considered.

STEP 1—STRUCTURING THE PROBLEM

In this exercise, the first step is to structure the problem. The case-study scenario (a) stated the major issue (the chance of seroconverting), (b) defined the perspective (an individual's experiencing a needle-stick), (c) identified options (taking or not taking AZT), and (d) defined the time horizon (at least 6 months).

STEP 2—DEVELOPING A DECISION TREE

Next, Williams constructs a decision tree, beginning with two initial arms (Figure C.1). Then, he identifies important outcomes. These outcomes are added to the decision tree (Figure C.2).

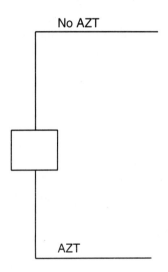

No AZT

AZT

Figure C.1 Two options.

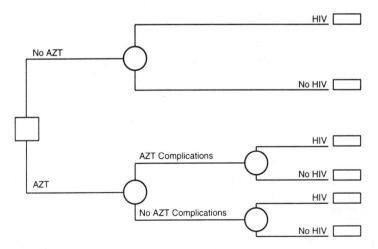

Figure C.2 Decision tree.

STEP 3—ASSIGNING PROBABILITIES

The next step is to assign probabilities for the four chance nodes:

    a. HIV infection without AZT treatment
    b. AZT-associated complications
    c. HIV infection with AZT treatment and complications
    d. HIV infection with AZT treatment and no complications

Once probabilities have been assigned to the branches at each of these four nodes, the other four probabilities can be calculated easily, because the sum of probabilities at each chance node must equal 1.0. For example, the probability of acquiring HIV in the absence of treatment with AZT is estimated to be 0.003; thus the probability of not acquiring HIV in the absence of treatment with AZT is $1.0 - 0.003$ or 0.997. Probabilities for the other outcomes in this example have been derived by soliciting expert opinion, since no data from published studies are available.

STEP 4—VALUING CONSEQUENCES

The next step involves the assignment of personal utilities for each of the outcomes in the decision tree. Williams uses a simple rank and scale method in his example, although more sophisticated methods could have been used (see Figure C.3).

STEP 5—AVERAGING-OUT-AND-FOLDING-BACK

Next, the expected values of the two choices at the decision node are calculated by averaging-out-and-folding-back. For example, the value or expected utility of 99.73 for the decision "No AZT" is derived as follows:

$$(0.003 \times 8.57) + (0.997 \times 100) = 99.73$$

This is illustrated in the full decision tree shown in Figure C.3

STEP 6—INTERPRETING RESULTS AND CONDUCTING SENSITIVITY ANALYSES

The final step is to interpret the results. Using the values assigned, the decision "No AZT" has the highest value and is the preferred decision. However, the decision maker may not be comfortable with this decision, especially since the estimates of probability and utility that go into the analysis are somewhat subjective.

    The solution to this problem is to do a sensitivity analysis, in which the uncertain values are allowed to vary through reasonable ranges in repeated

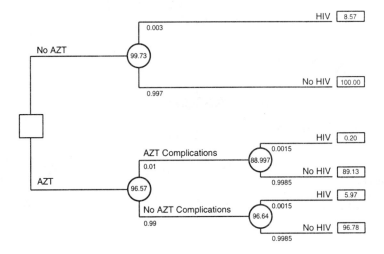

Figure C.3 Full decision tree.

calculations to see whether doing so changes the relationship of the values at the decision node. A threshold analysis is also done to determine the probability values at which the relationship is reversed.

When Williams did this, he found that the relationship could be reversed in the following situations:

a. When the risk of HIV infection is increased to at least 0.07
b. When the utility of AZT without complications and no HIV is increased to 100

However, he found that the relationship was not reversed in the following situations:

a. When the probability of AZT complications was reduced to zero
b. When the protective value of AZT was increased tenfold from its baseline value
c. When the utility of AZT with complications and no HIV was increased to 100

Thus Williams determined that the decision was relatively robust, i.e, the decision with the greatest value (the preferred decision) would change only by assuming probabilities and utilities that are very unlikely to be true.

APPENDIX D
Assessing the Effectiveness
of Prevention: A Case Study

HAN CHOI
PHAEDRA A. SHAFFER

Disease XYZ is a hypothetical infectious disease of viral origin that has been identified as a major public health problem in the United States. Approximately 129,000 cases of Disease XYZ occur each year, with an estimated associated cost of $1.07 billion to the health-care system. Clinically, Disease XYZ leads to multiple outcomes, ranging from a self-limited illness with full recovery to rapid multiorgan failure resulting in death within 1 month of infection. As a result, this disease leads to approximately 2,580 deaths each year and leaves an estimated 3,870 persons permanently disabled. The viral pathogen responsible for Disease XYZ was first isolated in 1980. To date, attempts to find an effective treatment have failed.

The disease is transmitted most commonly through sexual intercourse via exchange of bodily fluids. Another proven mode of transmission is through respiratory secretions and droplet nuclei. Respiratory transmission occurs much less frequently, however, as the inoculum that is required for infection is very large and would only be present after prolonged exposure to an infected person in a confined space. Thus persons in a high-risk category for Disease XYZ are those who have multiple sexual partners and practice unprotected sex, tissue-transplant recipients, recipients of infected blood, and persons exposed to human contaminants of persons infected with Disease XYZ (e.g., health-care workers). Also, family members, classmates, or other close contacts of infected persons are also considered to be at higher risk because of their prolonged or repeated contact with infected individuals.

Once a person is infected with the virus that causes Disease XYZ, a number of clinical outcomes may occur. Disease XYZ results in certain symptoms that appear by the end of the 2- to 5-day incubation period and allow for a relatively easy presumptive diagnosis based on clinical appearance. These symptoms consist of a petechial malar rash that lasts for 1 week and resolves spontaneously;

mild fever and malaise; and a distinctive, permanent depigmentation of the skin limited to the lower torso. Disease XYZ is definitively diagnosed by serology test results. In 5% of infected persons, the disease progresses rapidly to a more severe stage characterized by multiorgan failure followed by permanent disability or death.

In 1991, a breakthrough in virus-cloning techniques led to the development of a relatively safe vaccine with approximately 95% efficacy to prevent Disease XYZ among susceptible individuals. Although the vaccine is relatively efficacious, the virus has been shown to be similar to influenza in that it is highly mutagenic and develops a new strain each year. Therefore, a new vaccine must be administered every year to combat the newly mutated strain of Disease XYZ. As with most vaccines, this vaccine is not effective as a therapeutic vaccine for persons already infected. The vaccine has been approved for use by the general population. This analysis is designed to determine the most cost-effective strategy for delivery of the vaccine. Two strategies for vaccine delivery have been proposed: universal vaccination of the U. S. population and a vaccination strategy targeted at the segment of the population with the greatest risk of Disease XYZ.

The first option is a universal vaccination strategy for the U. S. population, regardless of risk status. The vaccine would be administered by public and private health-care providers. In addition to a mass-media public-education program to encourage vaccinations, a targeted campaign to inform physicians and other health-care providers would be initiated. Universal vaccination, however, may lead to vaccination of people who are not at high risk for Disease XYZ.

The second option is a vaccination strategy that targets high-risk individuals. This strategy would be implemented by targeting health-care services used by members of the high-risk population, i.e., public, sexually transmitted disease clinics, drug rehabilitation clinics, and inpatient facilities where Disease XYZ is frequently diagnosed. This vaccination strategy includes passive contact-tracing of susceptible high-risk partners of an infected patient. Vaccinations would also be administered to high-risk individuals via their usual health-care providers. All persons at high risk for Disease XYZ seeking health-care services would be encouraged to be vaccinated. As proposed for the universal vaccination option, the high-risk strategy would include a public information campaign to encourage vaccination.

The two strategies are compared with a no-vaccination program option. This option is included to evaluate the universal and targeted vaccination strategies against a baseline comparator.

METHODOLOGY

The Model

This analysis uses a decision-analytic framework to assess the cost-effectiveness of the two vaccine strategies. The health outcome measured in this analysis is cases of Disease XYZ prevented. The comparative summary measure is the incremental cost per case of Disease XYZ prevented. The time frame for the vaccination program is 1 year. The analytic horizon includes all of the future costs associated with long-term health effects from cases of Disease XYZ that occur within the 1-year time frame. A societal perspective is taken, in which all costs and benefits associated with the vaccination strategies are included regardless of who pays and who receives them. From this perspective, the cost of the health outcomes is measured using the cost-of-illness approach, which includes direct medical and nonmedical costs, and costs associated with lost productivity. The analysis is also done from the health-care system perspective in which productivity losses are excluded.

The Decision Tree

The decision tree is shown in Figure 8.1. In this case, there are three branches that represent the three decision options. For each option, moving from left to right on the tree, there is a chance node that subdivides the population into high-risk and low-risk groups. Subsequent chance nodes represent vaccine compliance rates, vaccine efficacy, risk of disease and probability of disease outcomes; healthy, disability, and death. Probability estimates are entered for each of the chance nodes in the tree. The cost of all events that occur on the path from the decision node to the terminal node and value of the health outcome (disease = 1; no disease = 0) are entered as the values of the terminal node.

Epidemiologic Parameters

Table D.1 summarizes the epidemiologic parameters and probabilities in the decision tree.

Table D.1 Parameters and Probabilities

Parameters	Probability
Incidence of Disease XYZ in U.S. population	0.0005
Incidence of Disease XYZ in high-risk population	0.005
Incidence of Disease XYZ in low-risk population	0.00028
Percentage of U.S. population in high-risk group	0.05
Healthy outcome following Disease XYZ	0.95
Disabled due to Disease XYZ	0.03
Deceased due to Disease XYZ	0.02
Vaccine efficacy	0.95
Adverse reactions among vaccinated	0.00001
Compliance rate to vaccination: low-risk population	0.60
Compliance rate to vaccination: high-risk population	0.40

Incidence

Sample surveys have demonstrated that approximately 5% of the U. S. population engage in behavior that qualifies them as high risk for developing Disease XYZ. The incidence of Disease XYZ among the U. S. population is 5 cases per 10,000 persons (0.0005). Among the high-risk group the rate is estimated to be 5 cases per 1,000 persons (0.005). The incidence in the low-risk population is approximately 2.5 cases per 10,000 persons. Of the persons diagnosed as having Disease XYZ, 95% recover fully and 3% are left with a long-term disability. The mortality rate for Disease XYZ is 2%.

Efficacy

The vaccine for Disease XYZ is administered by one intramuscular injection, and is formulated to provide immunity for the current year's strain of the virus that causes Disease XYZ. The vaccine efficacy is approximately 95% across all age groups.

Compliance

The success or failure of the vaccination strategies largely depends on the compliance rate achieved among both the low-risk and the high-risk populations. The compliance rate is one of the most uncertain variables in the model and is based on estimates from coverage rates achieved by similar prevention strategies. In the baseline scenario, the annual compliance rate among the low-risk population is estimated at 0.6. Among the high-risk population is estimated at 0.4. A range of compliance rates is used in the sensitivity analysis.

Economic Parameters

All costs in this model are expressed in 1994 dollar values. A discount rate of 5% is used to discount costs of long-term health effects of Disease XYZ that will occur in future years. Cost variables are presented in Table D.2.

Cost of the Interventions

The costs of the vaccination program in the model include the cost of the vaccine, the administration of the vaccine, and the costs of the side effects from

Table D.2 Cost of the Intervention

VACCINE-ASSOCIATED COSTS	
Average cost per dose of vaccine	$5
Average cost of vaccine administration	$15
TOTAL	$20
VACCINE ADVERSE REACTION-ASSOCIATED COSTS	
Physician visits/case of adverse reaction	$35
Time lost from work (3 hr. @ $13/hr.)	$39
TOTAL	$74

the vaccine. The estimates for vaccine-associated costs are based on retail price data, government prices for vaccine, and data from the National Medical Expenditure Survey and the National Health Interview Survey. The government price of the vaccine is $2.50 per dose; the private sector price is $6.25 per dose, a weighted average cost of $5.00 per dose. The cost of a public clinic visit for vaccine administration is $10.00, and the cost of a private office visit for vaccine administration is $17.50, for a weighted average cost of $15.00 for vaccine administration. Data from national sample surveys indicate that approximately two-thirds of those in both the general and high-risk populations will receive the vaccine from the private sector. Thus the average cost of a vaccination for both the targeted and the universal vaccination strategies is $20.00. The cost of patient time and travel to obtain the vaccine is not included because data was not available.

The only adverse reaction associated with vaccination is a localized exfoliation of the skin at the site of vaccination. This localized reaction resolves spontaneously within 2–3 weeks. The adverse reaction occurs in association with 1 out of every 100,000 vaccinations, and all persons are at equal risk for this reaction. The only complication is the possibility of cellulitis if the site becomes infected. Thus one follow-up visit to a physician is usually required. The cost of an adverse reaction to the vaccine is $35 for a follow-up physician visit and $39 for 3 hours of lost work. The only other vaccine program cost is the cost of public service announcements and other vaccine-awareness campaigns. In a study taking the societal perspective, these costs would be included because they represent costs of the program, regardless of who pays them. For the purposes of this case study, however, these costs are not included in the analysis—nor are the additional costs to the program resulting from the passive contact-tracing protocol.

Cost-of-Illness:

The cost-of-illness estimates for the health outcomes were derived from data from the National Medical Expenditure Survey, the National Health Interview Survey, the published literature, and the productivity loss tables in Appendix I adjusted for annual increases in earnings. The costs of the health outcomes are presented in Table D.3.

For the healthy outcome after a self-limited illness, ambulatory care is the only medical cost, estimated at $200. This includes the cost of 2 physician visits, laboratory tests, and medication. The cost of lost productivity is based on an estimate of 7 days of morbidity. Using estimates of the value of an unspecified (work or weekend) day, productivity losses for a healthy outcome are $505. The total cost of a healthy outcome is $705.

The estimated medical costs of the permanent disability outcome include the initial hospitalization costs and the costs of long-term care for the debilitating effects of the chronic sequelae. The cost of an average inpatient stay of 2 weeks for acute illness is $28,000. Survival of an episode of Disease XYZ severe enough to warrant inpatient treatment invariably results in lifetime disability for the patient. The annual medical and nonmedical cost includes $375 for 8 to 10

Table D.3   Cost of the Health Outcome

Health Outcome	Medical and Nonmedical Costs	Productivity Losses	Total Cost
Healthy	$200 - Ambulatory care	$505 (7 days)	$705
Disabled	$233,907 (Total medical & nonmedical) $28,000 - Hospitalization $205,907 - Total lifetime Disability costs; Annual costs include: $375 physician $4,800 therapy $4,000 nonmed.	$604,018 (Lifetime)	$837,925
Death	$56,000 - Hospitalization	$604,018 (Lifetime)	$660,018

physician visits per year, rehabilitative therapy at an annual cost of $4,800, and $4,000 for other nonmedical costs (including home health aides). Assuming a range in the age at which disability occurs, the average present value of lifetime medical and nonmedical disability costs, discounted at 5%, is $205,907.

Because of the chronic and incapacitating nature of this health outcome, it is assumed that a person disabled by Disease XYZ is unable to work again. Thus the average present value of lifetime productivity losses, adjusted for age and gender, and discounted at 5%, is $604,018.

The medical costs of the mortality outcome are an estimated $56,000, assuming that death occurs within 4 weeks of diagnosis and the patient requires hospitalization throughout that period. The estimate of lost productivity for mortality is the same as with disability.

Incremental Cost-Effectiveness Ratios
The summary measure produced by this analysis is the incremental cost-effectiveness ratio. This ratio reports the incremental impact of investment in the next most effective program, measured as cases of Disease XYZ prevented. The ratio is expressed as the additional cost per additional case of Disease XYZ prevented.

Sensitivity Analysis
The purpose of sensitivity analysis is to determine the effect of changes in parameter estimates on the decision result. Sensitivity analyses are performed either to answer specific policy questions or when uncertainty exists about the parameter estimates. The range of variables used in the sensitivity analyses for this study are based on medical literature, confidence intervals from meta-

analytic studies, and best-judgment estimates by experts in the field. Sensitivity analyses can be performed one variable at a time or several parameters can be varied simultaneously.

The following variables are considered for the sensitivity analyses in this study: vaccine efficacy, compliance with the vaccination program, the cost of the vaccine and administration, and the discount rate. Because of the number of variables for which uncertainty exists, we created "best-case" and "worst-case" scenarios to provide a realistic range of the impact that these vaccination strategies would have on morbidity and mortality from Disease XYZ (Table D.4). The best-case scenario uses estimates that favor vaccination programs. The worst-case scenario uses estimates that favor a no-vaccination program.

RESULTS

The purpose of this case study was to determine the most cost-effective vaccine delivery strategy. After calculating expected costs and expected cases of Disease XYZ for the U. S. population, the respective vaccination strategies can be compared on the basis of the incremental cost of preventing a case of Disease XYZ.

The projected results for the societal perspective, which include medical and nonmedical costs and productivity losses, and the health-care system perspective, which includes only the medical and nonmedical costs, are given in Table D.5. Without a vaccination program scenario, there would be 129,000 cases of Disease XYZ, 3,970 permanent disabilities, and 2,580 deaths. The total cost of the disease would exceed $5 billion; $1 billion in medical and nonmedical costs and $4 billion in productivity losses.

A Disease XYZ vaccination program targeted at high-risk individuals would prevent 23,750 (18%) cases of Disease XYZ per year including 712 permanent

Table D.4   Parameters for Sensitivity Analysis

Parameters	Worst Case	Base	Best Case
Compliance: general population	0.50	0.60	0.70
Compliance: high-risk group	0.30	0.40	0.50
Vaccine efficacy	0.90	0.95	0.98
Average cost per dose of vaccine	$30	$20	$10
Incidence: general population	0.005	0.0005	0.0005
Incidence: high-risk group	0.005	0.005	0.005
Percentage population at high risk	0.05	0.05	0.05
Healthy outcome	0.95	0.95	0.95
Disabled outcome	0.03	0.03	0.03
Deceased outcome	0.02	0.02	0.02

Table D.5   Results for the U.S. Population ($ in millions)

Characteristic	Status Quo—No Program	Targeted Vaccination	Universal Vaccination
INTERVENTION COST	—	100	2,905
OUTCOMES COST			
Societal Perspective			
Healthy outcome	86	70	45
Disability	3,243	2,646	1,693
Death	1,703	1,390	889
Total outcome cost	5,032	4,106	2,627
Total Cost	5,032	4,206	5,532
Health Care System Perspective			
Healthy outcome	25	20	13
Disability	905	739	473
Death	144	118	75
Total outcome cost	1,074	877	561
Total Cost	1,074	977	3,466
CASES OF DISEASE			
Healthy outcome	122,550	99,987	63,977
Disability	3,870	3,158	2,021
Death	2,580	2,105	1,347
Total cases	129,000	105,250	67,345

disabilities and 475 deaths. The targeted vaccination program would cost $100 million per year. However, the costs of the disease are reduced by $926 million; $197 million of the savings are medical and nonmedical costs and $729 million are productivity losses prevented. The net cost of the program from the societal perspective would be $4.2 billion, a savings of $826 million. The health-care system would save $97 million.

A universal Disease XYZ vaccination program would prevent an additional 37,905 (29%) cases, 1,137 permanent disabilities, and 758 deaths. This program would prevent 47% of the total cases that are projected to occur without a vaccination program. The cost of a universal vaccination program would be almost $3 billion. Medical and nonmedical costs are reduced by $316 million; productivity losses are reduced by $1.2 billion. Although the cost of the disease would be reduced by an additional $1.5 billion (compared with a targeted program), the $5.6 billion net cost of the program (from the societal perspective) exceeds the net cost of the two alternative options.

Incremental Cost-Effectiveness Ratios

The incremental cost-effectiveness ratios for the three strategies, ranked in order of effectiveness, are presented in Table D.6. From the societal perspec-

Table D.6   Cost-Effectiveness Ratios for Two Vaccination Strategies from
the Societal Perspective

	Total Cost (billions)	Additional Cost (Savings) (millions)[a]	Cases of Disease	Additional Cases Prevented[a]	Incremental Cost (Savings) per Case Prevented[b]
No Program	$5.032	—	129,000	—	—
Targeted Program	$4.206	($826)	105,250	23,750	($35,000)
Universal Program	$5.577	$1,371	67,345	37,905	$36,000

[a] Compared with next most effective program
[b] Rounded to the nearest thousand

tive, implementing a targeted vaccination program would save $35,000 per case
of Disease XYZ prevented. If the program was expanded to provide universal
vaccination, the additional 37,905 cases prevented would cost $36,000 each.

From the health-care system perspective, the targeted program would reduce
costs to the health-care system by $4,000 per case prevented, but expansion of
the program to universal coverage would cost the system an additional $67,000
per case.

Sensitivity Analyses

The results of the sensitivity analyses are shown in Table D.7. When estimates
are varied from the worst-case to the best-case scenario, the incremental cost

Table D.7   Sensitivity Analysis: CE Ratios[a]

Perspective/ Strategy	Best-Case Scenario	Base-Case Scenario	Worst-Case Scenario
Societal			
Targeted	($37,000)	($35,000)	($32,000)
Universal	($2,562)	$36,000	$80,000
Health-care system			
Targeted	($6,000)	($4,000)	($2,000)
Universal	$28,000	$67,000	$111,000

[a] Rounded to the nearest thousand

per case prevented for the targeted vaccination program, from both the societal
and the health-care system perspectives, always represents a savings. However,
the universal vaccination option only becomes less expensive than the other two
options in the best-case scenario, but only for the societal perspective. From the
health-care system perspective, the additional cost per case prevented with the
universal vaccination option is always greater than $28,000, even under the
best-case scenario. As expected, the programs' cost-effectiveness was most

sensitive to the price of the vaccine. When the vaccine price was reduced to $10, universal vaccination becomes a cost-saving strategy from the societal perspective. However, even at this price, the universal option would increase health-care-system costs by $1 billion annually. The cost-effectiveness of the two vaccination options was also sensitive to the vaccine compliance rate. Sensitivity analysis on the discount rate had little effect on the results of the analysis.

DISCUSSION

In this example, a cost-effectiveness analysis assists the policymaker by presenting information on specific decision options for addressing a preventable, public health problem. The results of the analysis indicate that a targeted vaccination program is the most cost-effective strategy for reducing the incidence of Disease XYZ in the U. S. population. From the societal perspective, the universal program is more effective in preventing cases of Disease XYZ but is an expensive option. As long as the cost of administering the program and the compliance rate meet the base-case projections, the targeted program is the optimal vaccination strategy. However, if the cost of the program is lower and the compliance rate is higher than projected, the universal vaccination program may be a more viable option if resources are available.

Policymakers may also be interested in the impact each option will have on the health-care system. This question was addressed by excluding productivity losses from the analysis. The results of this analysis from the health-care-system perspective indicate that the targeted vaccination program is the only strategy that decreases total health-care costs. Sensitivity analyses demonstrated that over a range of variable estimates, the universal program imposed a cost increase on the health-care system.

Although many more cases of Disease XYZ are prevented through universal vaccination, implementation costs are so high that the cost-effectiveness of the program is diminished. From the standpoint of the health-care system, decision makers must negotiate a trade-off between costs and the preventability of disease. Decision makers must also be informed that the intangible costs of the illness have not been included in this analysis. Thus, the trade-off between cost and effectiveness must also include the subjective valuation of pain and suffering and diminished quality of life.

Much depends on society's values and the amount of resources available. If society values a healthy life above all else, then decision makers may be willing to spend as much as necessary to prevent the most disease. In today's world, however, resources need to be used in the most effective way possible. Cost-effectiveness analyses are performed to assist policymakers to achieve that goal.

This case study illustrates the basic principles of an economic analysis by assessing the cost-effectiveness of two simplified vaccination strategies for a hypothetical disease, Disease XYZ. Although prevention effectiveness studies that address real-world problems involve other assumptions and techniques, the basic model and format of the decision tree are applicable and provide the framework necessary to identify real-world solutions.

APPENDIX E
Sources for Collecting Cost-of-Illness Data

Collecting reliable cost-of-illness data is one of the most difficult aspects of conducting an economic analysis. Data are often unavailable; data may not be generalizable to another population; or data do not reflect true economic costs. This appendix includes sources for collecting costs of illness and injury, including (a) literature reviews, (b) public-use tapes, (c) annually published materials, (d) miscellaneous journal articles, and (e) data collected by the private sector.

LITERATURE REVIEWS

The first step in a cost analysis is a literature review for published studies that assess similar health outcomes. In cases in which similar health outcomes have been studied, published studies may provide cost data that can be directly applied to a particular analysis. In other cases, a study of a similar (but not identical) health outcome may provide valuable data that can be extrapolated to fit the study design.

When using data from a published study, it is often helpful to use the same assumptions so the results of the various studies are comparable. For example, if a published study on the same health outcome uses the willingness-to-pay methodology, the same costs and methodology should also be used to maximize comparability.

There are several mechanisms by which to begin a thorough search of the literature. Data bases such as *Medline, BRS Colleague,* and *Dialog,* can be accessed from a national telecommunications network. Most academic libraries provide access to such networks.

Medline

MEDLINE is produced by the National Library of Medicine (NLM) and contains bibliographic citations from over 3,500 medical journals. Topics covered include medicine, nursing, dentistry, veterinary medicine, and preclinical sciences. Citations, dating back to 1966, are indexed by over 14,000 medical subject headings (MeSH), including health-care costs, cost-benefit analysis, and costs analysis. Over 80 subheadings, including economics, are also used. Most citations entered after 1975 contain abstracts.

BRS Colleague

Data bases that can be accessed through *BRS Colleague* include the following:

1. *ABI/INFORM*: The source for business and management information. Contains citations to more than 800 publications. Features full text of 100 of the most important journals. Covers such areas as economics and health care.
2. *Current Contents*: Includes the complete *Current Contents* data base, which includes the following subgroups: Agriculture, Biology & Environmental Sciences, Arts & Humanities, Clinical Medicine, Engineering, Technology & Applied Sciences, Life Sciences, Physical, Chemical & Earth Sciences, and Social & Behavioral Sciences.
3. *Health Periodicals Data Base*: A source of layperson-oriented abstracts; author abstracts; and full text on health, medicine, fitness, and nutrition. Providing timely and broad-based coverage of the entire health industry, the data base is designed to meet the research needs of business and health professionals as well as consumers.
4. *Health Planning and Administration:* An information resource for medical professionals, health-care managers, hospital administration, students, and librarians. Citations are taken from *MEDLINE* and additional health-related journals as selected. *MeSH* headings are used.
5. *Journal Watch:* A medical literature surveillance service that uses physician-editors to report on and summarize the most important new articles published in 20 leading journals. Journals include *JAMA, The New England Journal of Medicine, The Lancet, Annals of Internal Medicine, Journal of Infectious Diseases, Nature, Science, Cancer, Circulation, Pediatrics,* and *MMWR.*
6. *Social SciSearch:* Multidisciplinary data base covering the social sciences including economics and public health. Fully indexes more than 1,500 journals worldwide. Also contains relevant articles selected from approximately 3,100 additional journals in the natural, physical, and biomedical sciences.
7. *Wilson Social Sciences Index:* Comprehensive subject coverage includes community health and medical care, economics, planning and public administration, policy sciences.

Dialog

Some of the data bases that are available through *Dialog,* via the *Medical Connection,* are

1. *Agricola: Agricola* provides comprehensive information in the field of agriculture in its broadest sense. It includes references to materials indexed in the *Bibliography of Agriculture,* the *National Agriculture Library Catalog,* and the *Catalog of the Food and Nutrition Information and Education Resources Center (FNIC).* Abstracts are included for materials indexed by *FNIC* and by the *American Agricultural Economics Documentation Center (AAEDC).*
2. *Newsearch:* Provides front-page to back-page indexing of the *Christian Science Monitor,* the *New York Times,* the *Wall Street Journal,* the *Washington Post,* and the *Los Angeles Times,* and well as indexing over 370 popular American magazines, 660 law journals, and 6 law newspapers. Subject areas include Business and Economics, Health, Medicine, Environmental Issues, Science, Technology, and Agriculture.

CBA/CEA Bibliography

This bibliography of health-related articles on CBA and CEA has been published in *Medical Care* Supplement, July 1993, Vol. 31, No. 7. Subjects are cross-referenced by health condition and method. Over 3,200 CBA/CEA studies and reviews from 1979 through 1990 are included. References were identified from MEDLARS, CATLINE, a reference list of key articles identified in previous literature reviews, and lists obtained from leading health service researchers across the nation. The Centers for Disease Control and Prevention (CDC) has contracted for the update of this bibliography to 1994, to be made available by the end of 1995. In addition, health economic studies published between 1979 and 1994 pertaining to cost-of-illness, cost of intervention, and economic decision analyses methodology will be identified.

The bibliography will soon be available online from the CDC via the Internet.

PUBLIC-USE TAPES

After completing a literature search, the next step is to gather any data pertaining to the cost and health outcomes under analysis. There are several national data sources administered by federal agencies, such as the National Center for Health Statistics (NCHS) and the Health Care Financing Administration (HCFA), that provide aggregated data either on the state or national level. The following list comprises the most frequently used sources of raw, aggregated data.

National Hospital Discharge Survey (NHDS), NCHS

Provides information on patients discharged from short-stay hospitals in the United States. Data are available from 1970 to 1992. Surveys are conducted at a 1% sampling (approximately 400–500) of all short-stay hospitals in the United States. Variables include demographics, expected source of payment, discharge status, length of stay, hospital characteristics, and diagnostic and procedure codes. Data can be purchased from the National Technical Information Service (NTIS), (703) 487-4670. Prices range from $210 to $360 per tape, depending on the year.

National Medical Care Utilization and Expenditures Survey (NMCUES), NCHS

Between February 1980 and April 1981, NMCUES collected information from over 6,000 U. S. families, representing over 17,000 individuals. Data cover areas such as individual records for medical visits, dental visits, hospital stay, prescribed medicines, and the associated charges and payment sources for each. Data can be purchased from NTIS, (703) 487-4670. Cost is $820.

National Ambulatory Medical Care Survey (NAMCS), NCHS

Includes a probability sample of ambulatory medical encounters, covering non-hospital physician-patient encounters. The NAMCS data are available for 1973, 1975–81, 1985, and 1989–1991. Variables include date of visit, age, sex, race, ethnicity, reason for visit, source of payment, and diagnostic services. Data from 1973 to 1991 can be purchased from NTIS, (703) 487-4670. Data from 1992 can be purchased from NCHS, (301) 436-7132. Cost is $240 per tape.

National Mortality Followback Survey (NMFS), NCHS

Provides data on persons aged 25 years old and over who died in 1986. Variables include household composition, family income, and health care provided in the last year of life. Data can be purchased from NTIS, (703) 487-4670.

National Health Interview Survey (NHIS), NCHS

Implemented since 1957, NHIS provides data on self-reported illness. It involves a personal interview performed weekly of a sampling of U. S. households. Variables include restricted activity days, bed days, work/school lost days, physician visits, hospital episodes, and surgeries. Data on basic health and demographic questionnaires can be purchased from NTIS, (703) 487-4670. Data on NHIS current health topics can be purchased from Division of Health Interview Statistics, (301) 436-7085. Cost is approximately $200 per tape.

Medicare Data, HCFA

The Health Care Financing Administration (HCFA) sells public-use tapes on Medicare data that provide information on (a) utilization, (b) enrollment, (c) providers, (d) cost limits, (e) payment rates, and (f) cost reports on inpatients, capital, nursing facilities, and outpatients. Some examples of data files available are the following:

MEDPAR Files—The Medicare Provider Analysis and Review (MEDPAR) file contains records of hospital inpatient services. Available at the national and state levels.

Part B Provider Files—Contains claims submitted by a 5% sample of physicians and other providers of health-care services.

Medicaid Data, HCFA

Published state-by-state and available on an annual basis; provides aggregated data on the state level. HCFA also provides the Medicaid Statistical File, form HCFA-2082, Statistical Report on Medical Care: Eligibles, Recipients, Payments, and Services. This file reports Medicaid costs and utilization data that are submitted annually by states, territories, and the District of Columbia.

Public-use tapes, including both Medicare and Medicaid data, can be purchased from HCFA, (401) 597-5151.

ANNUALLY PUBLISHED MATERIAL

In addition to the public-use tapes, there are several publications that provide nationally aggregated data on an annual basis.

The DRG Handbook: Comparative Clinical and Financial Standards:

Provides (a) a complete charge breakdown and analysis of 53 major diagnosis-related groups (DRGs), (includes a detailed charge analysis providing cost data for ancillary services such as laboratory, radiology, medical supplies, and pharmacy); (b) summary information for all DRGs (includes average length of stay, and average total charge per discharge [$]); and (c) comparison group information for all major diagnostic categories (MDCs) (includes a regional and hospital-type breakdown of data).

The DRG Handbook is a good source of cost data only for specific types of studies—those with health outcomes that can be categorized into a DRG. In addition, the handbook assesses Medicare claims only, so one should be cautious in trying to interpolate data for all age groups. The DRG Handbook is published annually by HCIA and Ernst & Young, 1-800-568-3282. HCIA also produces annual publications on hospital inpatient charges, hospital admission rates, and length of stay (LOS).

Statistical Abstract of the U.S.

Published annually by the U.S. Department of Commerce, Economics and Statistics Administration, Bureau of the Census. The Abstract can be ordered from the Government Printing Office (GPO), (202) 793-3238, or from NTIS, (703) 487-4650. There are several tables that can provide data for an economic analysis:

- Medicare—Utilization and Charges. Includes percentage of covered charges reimbursed for hospital visits and percentage of covered charges reimbursed for physician visits.
- Consumer Price Indexes of Medical Care Prices. The medical-care commodities include prescription drugs and nonprescription drugs and medical supplies. The medical-care services include professional medical services, (i.e., physician charges, dental services, and eye care), and hospital and related services, (i.e., hospital rooms). See Appendix H.
- Average Cost to Community Hospitals per Patient.
- Average Cost to Community Hospitals per Patient, by State.
- Hospital Discharges and Days of Care, by Sex, Age, and Diagnosis. Diagnoses include diseases of heart, malignant neoplasms, pneumonia (all forms), fractures (all sites), and cerebrovascular diseases.
- Injury, Medical Care, Morbidity, and Mortality Costs, by Sex, Age, and Cause.
- Civilian Labor Force and Participation Rates by Race, Hispanic Origin, Sex, and Age.
- Employer Costs for Employee Compensation per Hour Worked, and by Industry.
- Median Money Income of Year-Round Full-Time Workers with Income, by Sex, Age, Race, and Hispanic Origin.

Health United States

Published annually by the U. S. Department of Health and Human Services, Centers for Disease Control and Prevention, National Center for Health Statistics, Hyattsville, Maryland. *Health United States* can be ordered from the Government Printing Office (GPO), (202) 793-3238, or from NTIS, (703) 487-4650. There are several tables that provide economic data:

- Hospital Expenses and Personnel and Average Annual Percent Change in Nonfederal Short-Stay hospitals.
- Nursing Home Average Monthly Charges per Resident and Percent of Residents, According to Selected Facility and Resident Characteristics.
- Hospital Utilization and Benefit Payments for Aged and Disabled Medicare Enrollees in Nonfederal Short-Stay Hospitals According to Geographic Division.
- Appendix I. Sources and Limitations of Data. Provides general overview of study design, methods of data collection, and reliability/validity of data. Also provides contact names for more information on each data set.

Hospital Statistics, Data from the American Hospital Association Annual Survey

Provides information on the average cost per hospital day, and the average length of a hospital stay. Published by the American Hospital Association, 1-800-242-2626.

OTHER DOCUMENTS AND JOURNAL ARTICLES

Finally, there are several documents and articles that provide excellent resources for assessing the cost of illness although they are not published on an annual basis. Some useful documents include:

Agency for Health Care Policy and Research's (AHCPR) *Clinical Classifications for Health Policy Research: Discharge Statistics by Principal Diagnosis and Procedure,* Provider Studies Research Note # 17, Pub. No. 93-0043, August 1993

The report presents statistics based on a 20% sample of discharges from the 1987 Hospital Cost and Utilization Project (HCUP). The report provides aggregated discharge data according to clinical condition or procedure. On the plus side, a compendium of such data for a national sample of hospital discharges has not been previously available. On the negative side, data represent charges for the hospitalization and do not necessarily reflect costs, nor are they synonymous with reimbursements. AHCPR publications can be ordered from their clearinghouse, 1-800-358-9295.

The Houston Center for Quality of Care and Utilization Studies *Database Sources for Research in Quality of Care and Utilization of Health Services, June 1992*

This center is a Veteran Health Services Research and Development Field Program designed to assess quality and outcomes to evaluate measures of utilization and cost. Their data base directory provides a comprehensive directory of data sources pertaining to quality and utilization from the federal government and private industry. Federal sources include data bases from (a) the Agency for Health Care Planning and Research (AHCPR), (b) the Bureau of the Census, (c) the Department of Defense (DOD), (d) the Environmental Protection Agency (EPA), (e) the Health Care Financing Administration (HCFA), and (f) the National Center for Health Statistics (NCHS). Private sources include (a) the American Hospital Association (AHA), (b) the American Medical Association (AMA), (c) the Health Insurance Association of America (HIAA), (d) the RAND Corporation, (e) the National Planning Data Corporation, and (f) various health maintenance organizations (HMOs). Each source includes a general description, the time period of available data, the variables included, and a contact name, address, and phone number. For more information, write Veterans' Affairs Medical Center, 2002 Holcombe Boulevard, Houston, TX 77030.

A list of selected journal articles that can provide useful information include:

- Gonzalez M (ed). *Socioeconomic characteristics of medical practice.* Chicago: The American Medical Association, 1992.
- Crane M. What your colleagues are charging. *Med Economics* Oct 19, 1992;69:20. *Medical Economics* survey shows fees in 14 specialties.

- Miller M, Welch WP. Physician charges in the hospital: exploring episodes of care for controlling volume growth. *Med Care* July 1992;30(7):630–45. This study reports physician services during the hospital stay and in the windows around the stay. Using 1987 data, this study presents average physician charges by type of service during (a) the hospital stay, and (b) 1-month windows before and after the stay. For all admissions, 85% of charges occur during the stay and 15% occur in the pre- and post-windows.
- American Hospital Association (AHA), 1991 National Hospital Panel Survey. Expenses per inpatient day. *Overview of entitlement programs: background material and data on programs within the jurisdiction of the Committee on Ways and Means.* Washington, D.C.: U.S. Congress, House of Representatives, 1992.
- Luce B, Elixhauser A. Estimating costs in the economic evaluation of medical technologies. *Int J Technology Assessment in Health Care* 1990;6:57–75.

PRIVATE SECTOR DATA AND CONSULTATION SOURCES

Another option for collecting cost-of-illness data is through a nongovernmental organization that owns or has access to large data bases containing information on costs. The advantages of using such a service are that (a) data collection for a specific study may not be required, and (b) a private organization may have access to information that would not ordinarily be available from public-use tapes. The disadvantages are that (a) purchasing private sector data bases can be costly, (b) some control over study design may be lost, and (c) data may be from selected populations. The following list provides a few of the organizations that are available for consultation.

HIAA—Health Insurance Association of America, (410) 576-9600. HIAA provides specific hospital charge data necessary for a particular study.

Blue Cross/Blue Shield. Center for Health Economics and Policy Research, (312) 440-6000. Provides data by illness category, at the transactional level. Looks at charges that are submitted and compares them to what is actually paid by BC/BS.

The Medstat Group, (313) 996-1180. Data base includes private-sector claims (both inpatient and outpatient) with interactive analytical software. Designed to help the health-care policymaker understand health-care costs and utilization patterns, levels, and trends in order to evaluate matters involving health benefits and policy evaluation. Software provides interactive access to other data bases such as Medicare and Medicaid.

The Codman Research Group, (603) 448-4044. Maintains a data base that includes discharges (by ICD-9 codes) from 16 states.

Battelle Human Affairs Research Center, (703) 528-6603. Provides contractual services in the area of economic analysis. Staff includes a multidisciplinary team of health economists, health and behavioral scientists, epidemiologists, health policy analysts, statisticians, and evaluation researchers.

National Perinatal Information Center, (401) 274-0650. Maintains a large
hospital discharge data base developed from annual discharge data of their
member hospitals. These data represent 1 million discharges. In addition, the
center has an extensive multistate data base that represents almost 40% of all
hospital discharges in the United States. This data base has transformed the
disparate configuration of seven state data bases into a uniform data base
ready for reporting. Although the center does not sell the data, the staff are
available for consultation and analysis services at a negotiated price.

Appendix F
Cost-to-Charge Ratios

Statewide Average Operating Cost-to-Charge Ratios for Urban and Rural Hospitals (case weighted) April 1994

State	Urban	Rural
Alabama	0.447	0.518
Alaska	0.515	0.801
Arizona	0.484	0.637
Arkansas	0.585	0.516
California	0.458	0.566
Colorado	0.549	0.619
Connecticut	0.574	0.596
Delaware	0.603	0.527
District of Columbia	0.533	N/A
Florida	0.462	0.464
Georgia	0.555	0.553
Hawaii	0.547	0.632
Idaho	0.599	0.667
Illinois	0.537	0.613
Indiana	0.615	0.677
Iowa	0.573	0.741
Kansas	0.549	0.702
Kentucky	0.541	0.573
Louisiana	0.506	0.561
Maine	0.688	0.605
Maryland	0.764	0.807
Massachusetts	0.702	0.602
Michigan	0.546	0.668
Minnesota	0.597	0.686
Mississippi	0.578	0.547
Missouri	0.498	0.555
Montana	0.553	0.659
Nebraska	0.559	0.711
Nevada	0.423	0.521
New Hampshire	0.610	0.644
New Jersey	0.691	N/A
New Mexico	0.549	0.556

(Continued)

Statewide Average Operating Cost-to-Charge Ratios for Urban and Rural Hospitals (case weighted) April 1994

State	Urban	Rural
New York	0.635	0.730
North Carolina	0.579	0.536
North Dakota	0.660	0.693
Ohio	0.616	0.656
Oklahoma	0.529	0.583
Oregon	0.601	0.663
Pennsylvania	0.469	0.598
Puerto Rico	0.554	0.876
Rhode Island	0.606	N/A
South Carolina	0.537	0.537
South Dakota	0.569	0.653
Tennessee	0.545	0.568
Texas	0.509	0.609
Utah	0.596	0.655
Vermont	0.619	0.616
Virginia	0.553	0.575
Washington	0.663	0.759
West Virginia	0.585	0.528
Wisconsin	0.655	0.705
Wyoming	0.616	0.760

Source: The Federal Register, Volume 59, No. 102, Friday, May 27, 1994, pages 27838–9.

Appendix G
Discount and Annuitization Tables

Present Value of $1, Discounted to the *n*th Year

n	0%	1%	2%	3%	4%	5%	6%	7%	8%	9%	10%
1	1.0000	0.9901	0.9804	0.9709	0.9615	0.9524	0.9434	0.9346	0.9259	0.9174	0.9091
2	1.0000	0.9803	0.9612	0.9426	0.9246	0.9070	0.8900	0.8734	0.8573	0.8417	0.8264
3	1.0000	0.9706	0.9423	0.9151	0.8890	0.8638	0.8396	0.8163	0.7938	0.7722	0.7513
4	1.0000	0.9610	0.9238	0.8885	0.8548	0.8227	0.7921	0.7629	0.7350	0.7084	0.6830
5	1.0000	0.9515	0.9057	0.8626	0.8219	0.7835	0.7473	0.7130	0.6806	0.6499	0.6209
6	1.0000	0.9420	0.8880	0.8375	0.7903	0.7462	0.7050	0.6663	0.6302	0.5963	0.5645
7	1.0000	0.9327	0.8706	0.8131	0.7599	0.7107	0.6651	0.6227	0.5835	0.5470	0.5132
8	1.0000	0.9235	0.8535	0.7894	0.7307	0.6768	0.6274	0.5820	0.5403	0.5019	0.4665
9	1.0000	0.9143	0.8368	0.7664	0.7026	0.6446	0.5919	0.5439	0.5002	0.4604	0.4241
10	1.0000	0.9053	0.8203	0.7441	0.6756	0.6139	0.5584	0.5083	0.4632	0.4224	0.3855
11	1.0000	0.8963	0.8043	0.7224	0.6496	0.5847	0.5268	0.4751	0.4289	0.3875	0.3505
12	1.0000	0.8874	0.7885	0.7014	0.6246	0.5568	0.4970	0.4440	0.3971	0.3555	0.3186
13	1.0000	0.8787	0.7730	0.6810	0.6006	0.5303	0.4688	0.4150	0.3677	0.3262	0.2897
14	1.0000	0.8700	0.7579	0.6611	0.5775	0.5051	0.4423	0.3878	0.3405	0.2992	0.2633
15	1.0000	0.8613	0.7430	0.6419	0.5553	0.4810	0.4173	0.3624	0.3152	0.2745	0.2394
16	1.0000	0.8528	0.7284	0.6232	0.5339	0.4581	0.3936	0.3387	0.2919	0.2519	0.2176
17	1.0000	0.8444	0.7142	0.6050	0.5134	0.4363	0.3714	0.3166	0.2703	0.2311	0.1978
18	1.0000	0.8360	0.7002	0.5874	0.4936	0.4155	0.3503	0.2959	0.2502	0.2120	0.1799
19	1.0000	0.8277	0.6864	0.5703	0.4746	0.3957	0.3305	0.2765	0.2317	0.1945	0.1635
20	1.0000	0.8195	0.6730	0.5537	0.4564	0.3769	0.3118	0.2584	0.2145	0.1784	0.1486
21	1.0000	0.8114	0.6598	0.5375	0.4388	0.3589	0.2942	0.2415	0.1987	0.1637	0.1351
22	1.0000	0.8034	0.6468	0.5219	0.4220	0.3418	0.2775	0.2257	0.1839	0.1502	0.1228
23	1.0000	0.7954	0.6342	0.5067	0.4057	0.3256	0.2618	0.2109	0.1703	0.1378	0.1117
24	1.0000	0.7876	0.6217	0.4919	0.3901	0.3101	0.2470	0.1971	0.1577	0.1264	0.1015
25	1.0000	0.7798	0.6095	0.4776	0.3751	0.2953	0.2330	0.1842	0.1460	0.1160	0.0923
26	1.0000	0.7720	0.5976	0.4637	0.3607	0.2812	0.2198	0.1722	0.1352	0.1064	0.0839
27	1.0000	0.7644	0.5859	0.4502	0.3468	0.2678	0.2074	0.1609	0.1252	0.0976	0.0763
28	1.0000	0.7568	0.5744	0.4371	0.3335	0.2551	0.1956	0.1504	0.1159	0.0895	0.0693
29	1.0000	0.7493	0.5631	0.4243	0.3207	0.2429	0.1846	0.1406	0.1073	0.0822	0.0630
30	1.0000	0.7419	0.5521	0.4120	0.3083	0.2314	0.1741	0.1314	0.0994	0.0754	0.0573
31	1.0000	0.7346	0.5412	0.4000	0.2965	0.2204	0.1643	0.1228	0.0920	0.0691	0.0521
32	1.0000	0.7273	0.5306	0.3883	0.2851	0.2099	0.1550	0.1147	0.0852	0.0634	0.0474
33	1.0000	0.7201	0.5202	0.3770	0.2741	0.1999	0.1462	0.1072	0.0789	0.0582	0.0431
34	1.0000	0.7130	0.5100	0.3660	0.2636	0.1904	0.1379	0.1002	0.0730	0.0534	0.0391

(Continued)

183

Present Value of $1, Discounted to the nth Year (*Continued*)

n	0%	1%	2%	3%	4%	5%	6%	7%	8%	9%	10%
35	1.0000	0.7059	0.5000	0.3554	0.2534	0.1813	0.1301	0.0937	0.0676	0.0490	0.0356
36	1.0000	0.6989	0.4902	0.3450	0.2437	0.1727	0.1227	0.0875	0.0626	0.0449	0.0323
37	1.0000	0.6000	0.4806	0.3350	0.2343	0.1644	0.1158	0.0818	0.0580	0.0412	0.0294
38	1.0000	0.6852	0.4712	0.3252	0.2253	0.1566	0.1092	0.0765	0.0537	0.0378	0.0267
39	1.0000	0.6784	0.4619	0.3158	0.2166	0.1491	0.1031	0.0715	0.0497	0.0347	0.0243
40	1.0000	0.6717	0.4529	0.3066	0.2083	0.1420	0.0972	0.0668	0.0460	0.0318	0.0221
41	1.0000	0.6650	0.4440	0.2976	0.2003	0.1353	0.0917	0.0624	0.0426	0.0292	0.0201
42	1.0000	0.6584	0.4353	0.2890	0.1926	0.1288	0.0865	0.0583	0.0395	0.0268	0.0183
43	1.0000	0.6519	0.4268	0.2805	0.1852	0.1227	0.0816	0.0545	0.0365	0.0246	0.0166
44	1.0000	0.6454	0.4184	0.2724	0.1780	0.1169	0.0770	0.0509	0.0338	0.0226	0.0151
45	1.0000	0.6391	0.4102	0.2644	0.1712	0.1113	0.0727	0.0476	0.0313	0.0207	0.0137
46	1.0000	0.6327	0.4022	0.2567	0.1646	0.1060	0.0685	0.0445	0.0290	0.0190	0.0125
47	1.0000	0.6265	0.3943	0.2493	0.1583	0.1009	0.0647	0.0416	0.0269	0.0174	0.0113
48	1.0000	0.6203	0.3865	0.2420	0.1522	0.0961	0.0610	0.0389	0.0249	0.0160	0.0103
49	1.0000	0.6141	0.3790	0.2350	0.1463	0.0916	0.0575	0.0363	0.0230	0.0147	0.0094
50	1.0000	0.6080	0.3715	0.2281	0.1407	0.0872	0.0543	0.0339	0.0213	0.0134	0.0085
51	1.0000	0.6020	0.3642	0.2215	0.1353	0.0831	0.0512	0.0317	0.0197	0.0123	0.0077
52	1.0000	0.5961	0.3571	0.2150	0.1301	0.0791	0.0483	0.0297	0.0183	0.0113	0.0070
53	1.0000	0.5902	0.3501	0.2088	0.1251	0.0753	0.0456	0.0277	0.0169	0.0104	0.0064
54	1.0000	0.5843	0.3432	0.2027	0.1203	0.0717	0.0430	0.0259	0.0157	0.0095	0.0058
55	1.0000	0.5785	0.3365	0.1968	0.1157	0.0683	0.0406	0.0242	0.0145	0.0087	0.0053
56	1.0000	0.5728	0.3299	0.1910	0.1112	0.0651	0.0383	0.0226	0.0134	0.0080	0.0048
57	1.0000	0.5671	0.3234	0.1855	0.1069	0.0620	0.0361	0.0211	0.0124	0.0074	0.0044
58	1.0000	0.5615	0.3171	0.1801	0.1028	0.0590	0.0341	0.0198	0.0115	0.0067	0.0040
59	1.0000	0.5560	0.3109	0.1748	0.0989	0.0562	0.0321	0.0185	0.0107	0.0062	0.0036
60	1.0000	0.5504	0.3048	0.1697	0.0951	0.0535	0.0303	0.0173	0.0099	0.0057	0.0033
61	1.0000	0.5450	0.2988	0.1648	0.0914	0.0510	0.0286	0.0161	0.0091	0.0052	0.0030
62	1.0000	0.5396	0.2929	0.1600	0.0879	0.0486	0.0270	0.0151	0.0085	0.0048	0.0027
63	1.0000	0.5343	0.2872	0.1553	0.0845	0.0462	0.0255	0.0141	0.0078	0.0044	0.0025
64	1.0000	0.5290	0.2816	0.1508	0.0813	0.0440	0.0240	0.0132	0.0073	0.0040	0.0022
65	1.0000	0.5237	0.2761	0.1464	0.0781	0.0419	0.0227	0.0123	0.0067	0.0037	0.0020
66	1.0000	0.5185	0.2706	0.1421	0.0751	0.0399	0.0214	0.0115	0.0062	0.0034	0.0019
67	1.0000	0.5134	0.2653	0.1380	0.0722	0.0380	0.0202	0.0107	0.0058	0.0031	0.0017
68	1.0000	0.5083	0.2601	0.1340	0.0695	0.0362	0.0190	0.0100	0.0053	0.0029	0.0015
69	1.0000	0.5033	0.2550	0.1301	0.0668	0.0345	0.0179	0.0094	0.0049	0.0026	0.0014
70	1.0000	0.4983	0.2500	0.1263	0.0642	0.0329	0.0169	0.0088	0.0046	0.0024	0.0013
71	1.0000	0.4934	0.2451	0.1226	0.0617	0.0313	0.0160	0.0082	0.0042	0.0022	0.0012
72	1.0000	0.4885	0.2403	0.1190	0.0594	0.0298	0.0151	0.0077	0.0039	0.0020	0.0010
73	1.0000	0.4837	0.2356	0.1156	0.0571	0.0284	0.0142	0.0072	0.0036	0.0019	0.0010
74	1.0000	0.4789	0.2310	0.1122	0.0549	0.0270	0.0134	0.0067	0.0034	0.0017	0.0009
75	1.0000	0.4741	0.2265	0.1089	0.0528	0.0258	0.0126	0.0063	0.0031	0.0016	0.0008
76	1.0000	0.4694	0.2220	0.1058	0.0508	0.0245	0.0119	0.0058	0.0029	0.0014	0.0007

Annuitization Factor[a]

n^b	1%	2%	3%	4%	5%	6%	7%	8%	9%	10%
1	0.9901	0.9804	0.9709	0.9615	0.9524	0.9434	0.9346	0.9259	0.9174	0.9091
2	1.9704	1.9416	1.9135	1.8861	1.8594	1.8334	1.8080	1.7833	1.7591	1.7335
3	2.9410	2.8839	2.8286	2.7751	2.7232	2.6730	2.6243	2.5771	2.5313	2.4869
4	3.9020	3.8077	3.7171	3.6299	3.5460	3.4651	3.3872	3.3121	3.2397	3.1699
5	4.8534	4.7135	4.5797	4.4518	4.3295	4.2124	4.1002	3.9927	3.8897	3.7908
6	5.7955	5.6014	5.4172	5.2421	5.0757	4.9173	4.7665	4.6229	4.4859	4.3553
7	6.7282	6.4720	6.2303	6.0021	5.7864	5.5824	5.3893	5.2064	5.0330	4.8684
8	7.6517	7.3255	7.0197	6.7327	6.4632	6.2098	5.9713	5.7466	5.5348	5.3349
9	8.5660	8.1622	7.7861	7.4353	7.1078	6.8017	6.5152	6.2469	5.9952	5.7590
10	9.4713	8.9826	8.5302	8.1109	7.7217	7.3601	7.0236	6.7101	6.4177	6.1446
11	10.3676	9.7868	9.2526	8.7605	8.3064	7.8869	7.4987	7.1390	6.8052	6.4951
12	11.2551	10.5753	9.9540	9.3851	8.8633	8.3838	7.9427	7.5361	7.1607	6.8137
13	12.1337	11.3484	10.6350	9.9856	9.3936	8.8527	8.3577	7.9038	7.4869	7.1034
14	13.0037	12.1062	11.2961	10.5631	9.8986	9.2950	8.7455	8.2442	7.7862	7.3667
15	13.8651	12.8493	11.9379	11.1184	10.3797	9.7122	9.1079	8.5595	8.0607	7.6061
16	14.7179	13.5777	12.5611	11.6523	10.8378	10.1059	9.4466	8.8514	8.3126	7.8237
17	15.5623	14.2919	13.1661	12.1657	11.2741	10.4773	9.7632	9.1216	8.5436	8.0216
18	16.3983	14.9920	13.7535	12.6593	11.6896	10.8276	10.0591	9.3719	8.7556	8.2014
19	17.2260	15.6785	14.3238	13.1339	12.0853	11.1581	10.3356	9.6036	8.9501	8.3649
20	18.0456	16.3514	14.8775	13.5903	12.4622	11.4699	10.5940	9.8181	9.1285	8.5136
21	18.8570	17.0112	15.4150	14.0292	12.8212	11.7641	10.8355	10.0168	9.2922	8.6487
22	19.6604	17.6580	15.9369	14.4511	13.1630	12.0416	11.0612	10.2007	9.4424	8.7715
23	20.4558	18.2922	16.4436	14.8568	13.4886	12.3034	11.2722	10.3711	9.5802	8.8832
24	21.2434	18.9139	16.9355	15.2470	13.7986	12.5504	11.4693	10.5288	9.7066	8.9847
25	22.0232	19.5235	17.4131	15.6221	14.0930	12.7834	11.6536	10.6748	9.8226	9.0770

[a] See chapter 6

[b] n = Length of capital life

Appendix H
Consumer Price Index

Consumer Price Index, for All Items and the Medical-Care
Component, 1960 to 1994

	All Items	Med-ical Care	Medical-Care Services				Hosp. Room	Medical Care Com-modities
			Total	Professional Services				
				Total	Phys.	Dental		
1960	29.6	22.3						
1965	31.5	25.2						
1970	38.8	34.0	32.3	37.0	34.5	39.2	23.6	46.5
1975	53.8	47.5	46.6	50.8	48.1	53.2	38.3	53.3
1980	82.4	74.9	74.8	77.9	76.5	78.9	68.0	75.4
1981	90.9	82.9	82.8	85.9	84.9	86.5	78.1	83.7
1982	96.5	92.5	92.6	93.2	92.9	93.1	90.4	92.3
1983	99.6	100.6	100.7	99.8	100.1	99.4	100.6	100.2
1984	103.9	106.8	106.7	107.0	107.0	107.5	109.0	107.5
1985	107.6	113.5	113.2	113.5	113.3	114.2	115.4	115.2
1986	109.6	122.0	121.9	120.8	121.5	120.6	122.3	122.8
1987	113.6	130.1	130.0	128.8	130.4	128.8	131.1	131.0
1988	118.3	138.6	138.3	137.5	139.8	137.5	143.3	139.9
1989	124.0	149.3	148.9	146.4	150.1	146.1	158.1	150.8
1990	130.7	162.8	162.7	156.1	160.8	155.8	175.4	163.4
1991	136.2	177.0	177.1	165.7	170.5	167.4	191.9	176.8
1992	140.3	190.1	190.5	175.8	181.2	178.7	208.7	188.1
1993	144.5	201.4	202.9	184.7	191.3	188.1	226.4	195.0
1994	149.7	215.3	218.2	196.0	203.1	201.4	244.3	202.9

Source: Statistical Abstract of the U.S., 1994, Tables No. 163: Consumer Price Indexes of Medical Care Prices: 1970 to 1993; and 756: Consumer Price Indexes, by Major Groups: 1960 to 1993; U.S. Bureau of Labor Statistics, *CPI Detailed Report*, January 1995; *Monthly Labor Review* and *Handbook of Labor Statistics*, periodic.

Appendix I
Productivity Loss Tables

TABLES I.1a, I.1b, I.1c

Disaggregated income data (by gender) were obtained from Dorothy P. Rice and Wendy Max, School of Nursing, University of California, San Francisco. Their sources include the following:

1. Population: National Center for Health Statistics, *Vital Statistics of the United States, 1989*, Volume II, Section 6. U. S. Department of Health and Human Services, Public Health Service, Centers for Disease Control and Prevention, Table 6–1.
2. Proportion of population with earnings and not in labor force and keeping house: U. S. Department of Labor, Bureau of Labor Statistics, *Employment and earnings*, January 1991. Table 3, "Employment status of the civilian noninstitutional population by age, sex, and race," page 164.
3. Annual mean earnings: U.S. Bureau of the Census, *Current population reports*, Series P-60, No. 180, Table 30, "Mean earnings, Year-round Fulltime workers." Adjusted by factor of 1.1734 to include fringe benefits. Age groups 15-24 and 75+ disaggregated using factors.
4. Annual Mean Value of Housekeeping Services: 1987 values for housekeeping services from Douglas J, Kenney G, Miller T. Which estimates of household production are best, *J Forensic Economics* December 1990; 4(1):25–45. These numbers were updated to 1990 using the percentage change in compensation per hour in the business sector from *Employment and Earnings*, U. S. Department of Commerce, Bureau of Labor Statistics, March, 1991.

Data Were Aggregated by Sex to Eliminate Any Bias

Data do not include proportion of the population unemployed. For example, the labor force population is the proportion of the population with earnings. The nonlabor force population is the proportion of the population without earnings

Table I.1a Total for Males and Females, 1990 Data

Age in Years	Labor Force				Nonlabor Force		
	Proportion of Total Population	Annual Mean Earnings ($)	Annual Mean Value of Hskeep ($)	Annual Mean Earnings w/Value of Hskeep ($)	Proportion of Total Population	Annual Mean Value of Hskeep ($)	Weighted Average Earnings of Labor & Nonlabor($)
Under 1	0	0	0	0	0	0	0
1-4	0	0	0	0	0	0	0
5-9	0	0	0	0	0	0	0
10-14	0	0	0	0	0	0	0
15-19	0.432	13,694	3,675	17,369	0.029	10,795	16,956
20-24	0.7792	19,128	4,590	23,718	0.0805	11,854	22,608
25-29	0.8372	26,911	5,701	32,612	0.1071	13,850	30,484
30-34	0.8388	31,300	6,540	37,840	0.1144	15,193	35,123
35-39	0.8506	36,259	6,908	43,167	0.1048	15,562	40,140
40-44	0.856	38,462	6,885	45,347	0.1203	15,253	41,639
45-49	0.8334	39,006	6,571	45,577	0.1072	14,582	42,044
50-54	0.7751	37,284	6,511	43,795	0.1416	14,561	39,278
55-59	0.6704	36,515	6,513	43,027	0.1807	14,593	36,991
60-64	0.4491	35,011	6,468	41,479	0.2287	14,580	32,404
65-69	0.2112	32,805	6,443	39,248	0.2652	14,228	25,321
70-74	0.1137	32,734	4,502	37,235	0.2967	10,121	17,631
75-79	0.0606	25,335	3,031	28,366	0.29	6,872	10,588
80-84	0.0346	21,482	1,732	23,214	0.2798	3,999	6,116
85 & Over	0.0191	17,058	1,047	18,105	0.2587	2,269	3,360

Annual Mean Earnings Weighted by Age: $23,582
Value of a Lost Work Day: $94
Value of an Unspecified Day: $65

Table I.1b Females, 1990

	Labor Force				Nonlabor Force		
Age in Years	Proportion of Total Population	Annual Mean Earnings ($)	Annual Mean Value of Hskeep ($)	Annual Mean Earnings w/Value of Hskeep ($)	Proportion of Total Population	Annual Mean Value of Hskeep ($)	Weighted Average Earnings of Labor & Nonlabor($)
Under 1	0	0	0	0	0	0	0
1–4	0	0	0	0	0	0	0
5–9	0	0	0	0	0	0	0
10–14	0	0	0	0	0	0	0
15–19	0.418	13,507	5,267	18,774	0.0538	11,199	17,910
20–24	0.716	17,890	6,101	23,991	0.155	12,034	21,863
25–29	0.738	23,961	8,064	32,025	0.2081	13,997	28,060
30–34	0.734	26,086	9,421	35,507	0.2216	15,354	30,834
35–39	0.755	28,081	9,813	37,894	0.2018	15,744	33,222
40–44	0.776	29,322	9,476	38,798	0.2313	15,408	33,427
45–49	0.748	28,124	8,795	36,919	0.205	14,726	32,145
50–54	0.669	22,637	8,795	35,432	0.2682	14,726	29,507
55–59	0.553	25,540	8,786	34,326	0.3404	14,719	26,855
60–64	0.355	24,370	8,786	33,156	0.4231	14,719	23,131
65–69	0.17	22,794	8,566	31,360	0.48	14,351	18,800
70–74	0.082	24,721	6,099	30,820	0.5182	10,218	13,033
75–79	0.04	17,613	4,148	21,761	0.4816	6,948	8,084
80–84	0.02	14,887	2,410	17,297	0.4385	4,037	4,615
85 & Over	0.013	12,589	1,364	13,953	0.3672	2,285	2,684

Annual Mean Earnings Weighted by Age: $18,983
Value of a Lost Work Day: $76
Value of an Unspecified Day: $52

Table I.1c Males, 1990

Age in Years	Labor Force				Nonlabor Force		Weighted Average Earnings of Labor & Nonlabor($)
	Proportion of Total Population	Annual Mean Earnings ($)	Annual Mean Value of Hskeep ($)	Annual Mean Earnings w/Value of Hskeep ($)	Proportion of Total Population	Annual Mean Value of Hskeep ($)	
Under 1	0	0	0	0	0	0	0
1–4	0	0	0	0	0	0	0
5–9	0	0	0	0	0	0	0
10–14	0	0	0	0	0	0	0
15–19	0.446	13,870	2,175	16,045	0.004	5,330	15,950
20–24	0.843	20,190	3,294	23,484	0.0052	6,450	23,380
25–29	0.938	29,270	3,811	33,081	0.0045	6,965	32,956
30–34	0.946	35,436	4,255	39,691	0.0047	7,410	39,531
35–39	0.949	42,961	4,527	47,488	0.0048	7,683	47,288
40–44	0.939	46,307	4,661	50,968	0.005	7,817	50,739
45–49	0.923	48,258	4,680	52,938	0.006	7,836	52,714
50–54	0.888	45,818	4,680	50,498	0.007	7,836	50,164
55–59	0.798	44,783	4,800	49,583	0.007	7,956	49,221
60–64	0.555	42,667	4,800	47,467	0.01	7,956	46,768
65–69	0.26	40,549	4,800	45,349	0.0111	7,956	43,818
70–74	0.154	38,171	3,418	41,589	0.0144	5,664	38,517
75–79	0.09	30,220	2,324	32,544	0.0173	3,852	27,918
80–84	0.059	25,202	1,350	26,552	0.0158	2,238	21,416
85 & Over	0.033	21,040	764	21,804	0.0132	1,267	15,936

Annual Mean Earnings Weighted by Age: $30,977
Value of a Lost Work Day: $124
Value of an Unspecified Day: $85

that are keeping house; therefore, their productive value is related to the value of their housekeeping. The data do not include the nonlabor force population that are not keeping house. This segment of the population would include those individuals who cannot care for themselves (i.e., children under age 15 and persons in institutions) and who neither work in the labor market nor work at home. Their productive value in terms of potential earnings would be $0.

Data Were Aggregated Across Age Groups to Eliminate Any Bias

The value of a lost work day is $94 (1990 dollars). It is the average annual earnings of an individual, weighted by age and sex ($23,582 divided by the number of days a full-time wage earner works—250 days). The value of an unspecified day (work or other) is $65 (1990 dollars), ($23,582 divided by 365 days) and includes leisure time lost on the nonworking days due to morbidity. For example, if an illness causes 2 weeks of morbidity, but it is unknown whether those days were work days or weekend days, morbidity is assessed at $65 per day to account for the work and nonwork days lost due to illness. If the actual number of work days lost is known, then morbidity would be assessed at $94 per workday.

NOTE: The values reported are based on 1990 earnings. Values should be adjusted to the appropriate year. See chapter 6.

TABLE I.2

Data Used from Table I.1 to Calculate Table I.2

The data in Table I.2 represent the productive population, i.e., those in the labor force with earnings and those not in the labor force keeping house. If the segment of the population that is unproductive had been included, the expected future lifetime earnings would be considerably lower, especially for the youngest and oldest age groups.

The lifetime earnings reported in Table I.2 are based on two assumptions: a 1% annual growth in productivity and a 75-year life expectancy. For ages ⟩ 74, the average annual mean earnings (undiscounted) of a 75-year-old person were used.

To obtain the weighted average lifetime income by age reported in the last row of Table I.2, 1990 population data were obtained from the *Statistical Abstract of the United States: 1993,* (113th edition) U. S. Bureau of the Census, Washington, D.C., 1993: Table 14 and Table 47.

Table I.2 Present Value of Expected Future Lifetime Earnings and Housekeeping Services According to Age*($)

Age Group	Discount Rate										
	0%	1%	2%	3%	4%	5%	6%	7%	8%	9%	10%
<1	3,029,313	1,913,683	1,242,076	827,514	565,176	395,077	282,163	205,509	152,363	114,782	87,721
1-4	2,955,068	1,913,683	1,273,126	869,299	608,410	435,774	318,856	237,899	180,657	139,384	109,083
5-9	2,825,774	1,913,683	1,330,889	949,627	694,288	519,293	396,647	308,826	244,649	196,848	160,606
10-14	2,688,627	1,913,683	1,398,092	1,047,448	803,710	630,597	508,641	412,122	342,024	288,175	246,104
15-19	2,524,891	1,879,771	1,434,100	1,120,070	894,405	729,079	605,660	511,844	439,290	382,260	336,742
20-24	2,308,971	1,783,687	1,407,654	1,133,738	930,736	777,721	660,473	559,196	497,056	439,220	392,223
25-29	2,071,738	1,654,895	1,346,225	1,114,203	937,193	800,178	692,615	607,017	538,009	481,683	435,170
30-34	1,814,140	1,493,197	1,247,732	1,057,608	908,504	790,137	695,051	617,786	554,316	501,623	457,442
35-39	1,545,788	1,307,548	1,119,602	969,788	849,147	751,026	670,443	603,641	547,759	500,606	460,488
40-44	1,273,008	1,103,850	966,337	853,624	760,487	682,914	617,804	552,745	515,847	475,622	440,888
45-49	1,008,338	894,845	739,845	719,818	651,984	594,136	544,509	501,689	464,537	432,127	403,707
50-54	760,764	690,157	629,328	576,678	530,897	490,910	455,831	424,926	397,585	373,301	351,648
55-59	537,692	498,341	463,471	432,470	404,821	380,085	357,887	337,908	319,874	303,549	288,732
60-64	341,056	322,560	305,709	290,324	276,250	263,349	251,500	240,598	230,548	221,266	212,679
65-69	181,120	174,706	168,698	163,063	157,772	152,799	148,120	143,713	139,557	135,634	131,929
70-74	64,514	63,481	62,487	61,530	60,608	59,714	58,863	58,035	57,237	56,466	55,721
>74	10,588	10,588	10,588	10,588	10,588	10,588	10,588	10,588	10,588	10,588	10,588
All ages	1,688,595	1,271,174	985,299	790,440	648,603	544,160	465,662	404,691	356,964	318,760	287,682

*Assumes an annual growth in productivity of 1%

Age at death = 75

APPENDIX J
Measures of Attribution

RICHARD B. ROTHENBERG
ROBERT A. HAHN

In the early 1950s, when Levin described mathematically the proportion of lung cancer mortality associated with smoking, he set the stage for refining and further defining the magnitude of the effect of risk factors on public health problems.[1] His premise was simply that the magnitude of the effect of a given risk factor in causing a health problem in a population could be measured and described objectively. This process is called *attribution*. Since that first article, investigators have continued to describe variations in calculating attribution, depending on the risk factors and population involved (variously called *attributable risk, etiologic fraction, population-attributable risk*, or *attributable risk among exposed persons*), and in describing the effects of preventive interventions on a population (*prevented fraction*).

Formulas for calculating attribution in many types of studies have been derived, and means of adjustment for confounding factors have been established. A summary formula that permits both attribution and prevention to be estimated has been developed for situations in which a risk factor is not fully eliminated or a preventive measure is not fully instituted (the *impact fraction*). The concept of attribution has been further defined to allow differentiation of *excess fraction* (the fractional excess case load produced by an exposure), *incidence density fraction* (the difference in incidence related to a particular exposure), and *etiologic fraction* (the quantitative statement of the role of a particular risk factor).

These concepts and their application are far from simple and straightforward. However, the pressing need to be able to assess the effectiveness of prevention strategies in the context of public health practice has made it desirable for epidemiologists, health economists, and others to use the concept of attribution. The paradigm upon which attribution is based is not complex: it is simply that risk factors cause health problems and that removing those risk factors will diminish the incidence of the health problems.

The following sections describe in greater detail the relationships among risk factors, outcomes, and interventions.

ATTRIBUTABLE RISK

Definition and Derivation

New cases of a health problem in a population occur at a certain rate (called *incidence* here). The incidence in the total population, called I_t, reflects the rate of occurrence of the problem both among persons exposed, I_1, and among persons not exposed, I_0, to the risk factor being assessed. "Risk factors" are conditions or events that increase the likelihood of a specific outcome, e.g., disease. If one subtracts the incidence among persons not exposed to the risk factor from the total incidence, the remainder reflects the incidence of the health problem among persons exposed to the risk factor being studied, and the proportion of incidence that can be attributed to that risk factor is called the *attributable risk* (AR).

$$AR = \frac{(I_t - I_o)}{I_t} \tag{1}$$

The attributable risk will always be between 0 and 1. If the incidence of the health problem for the total population and for the group not exposed to the risk factor being studied are equal $(I_t = I_0)$, then none of the cases of the health problem can be attributed to the risk factor being studied, and $AR = 0$. If, on the other hand, all cases of the disease occur among persons who have been exposed to the risk factor being studied, and $I_0 = 0$, the health problem is completely attributable to the risk factor being studied, and $AR = 1$.

Because in the real world of public health practice, it is not usually possible to obtain reliable estimates of the incidence of a health problem in a particular population, Levin derived an algebraic expression for attributable risk in terms of the *prevalence of exposure* (i.e., the proportion of a population that is or has been exposed to a particular risk factor at some instant in time) and the *relative risk* (RR) that the health problem will occur among persons who have been exposed compared with those who have not (I_1/I_0), a ratio that may be known from studies of other populations. Total incidence in equation (1) is replaced by the weighted sum of incidence among exposed and unexposed persons, with the weights being, in order shown, the prevalence of exposure (P_1) and lack of exposure $(1 - P_1)$. That is, $I_t = (P_1)(I_1) + (1 - P_1)(I_0)$.

$$AR = \frac{(I_1)(P_1) + (I_0)(1 - P_1) - I_0}{(I_1)(P_1) + (I_0)(1 - P_1)} \tag{2}$$

When simplified (by dividing numerator and denominator by I_0), the equation becomes

$$AR = \frac{P_1(RR - 1)}{1 + P_1(RR - 1)} \tag{3}$$

Equation (3) is the one most familiar to epidemiologists, although it neglects situations where there are multiple exposures and confounding. It does, however, permit the investigator to assess the effects of a single exposure on an outcome, ignoring contributions of other exposures. The AR describes the proportion of a health problem that would not have occurred if no one had been exposed to the risk factor being assessed.

Attributable risk can also be expressed in terms of the proportion of persons who have the health problem (P_p) and have been exposed to the risk factor being studied rather than the proportion of the total population that has been exposed to that same risk factor:

$$AR = P_p \left[\frac{RR - 1}{RR} \right] \qquad (4)$$

Unlike equation (3), equation (4) allows the use of an adjusted relative risk (i.e., a relative risk for a factor that has been calculated in the presence of potential confounding by other factors).

Equation (3) may also be modified to consider the proportion of cases attributable to exposure among persons exposed. In this situation, the prevalence of exposure, P_1, is 1 and equation (3) is reduced to:

$$AR_e = \frac{RR - 1}{RR} \qquad (5)$$

Multiple Exposures

Many health outcomes may be caused by several distinct risk factors, and individuals may be exposed to more than one risk factor. In addition, some risk factor exposures may be stratified into levels, e.g., blood cholesterol levels < 200 mg, 200–239 mg, and >239 mg. In order to allow calculations of attributable risk in such situations, a more general expression has been derived in which total incidence is subdivided into many levels ($I_0, I_1, I_2, \ldots I_n$), where I_0 is the incidence among persons who have not been exposed at any level to any of the risk factors being assessed. For each incidence (I_i), there will be a corresponding prevalence of exposure (P_i) and a corresponding relative risk ($RR_i = I_i / I_0$), with $RR_0 = 1$. If there are n different risk factors and r of them are capable of coexisting, the total number of possible exposures is the sum of n risk factors taken r at a time, as r varies from 1 to n. (This summation is equivalent to 2^n.)

For multiple exposures or multiple levels of exposure (where n is the total number of distinct exposure strata), using the proportion of the total population in each exposure stratum, the joint AR (AR_j) becomes:

$$AR_j = \frac{\sum_{i=1}^{n} (P_i)(RR_i - 1)}{1 + \sum_{i=1}^{n} (P_i)(RR_i - 1)} \qquad (6)$$

Or, AR_j can be written in terms of the proportion of cases in each stratum of exposure:

$$AR_j = 1 - \sum_{i=1}^{n} \frac{(P_i)}{RR_i} \qquad (7)$$

where P_i is the proportion of all cases in stratum i and RR_i is the relative risk for that stratum.

The AR_j is determined by the schedule of joint exposures and their corresponding relative risks in the population. The contribution of any specific stratum i to the overall AR_j is $(P_i)(RR_i - 1)/[1 + \Sigma(P_i)(RR_i - 1)]$. This relationship is useful in determining the portion of the total AR_j that results from a single exposure configuration or a grouping of configurations.

The AR_j is conceptually and algebraically different from the AR that would be obtained by making the usually incorrect assumption that exposures are mutually exclusive (i.e., that no person is exposed to more than one risk factor) and adding the attributable risks for each exposure (AR_m). The AR_m is calculated by summing over equation (3):

$$AR_m = \sum_{i=1}^{n} \frac{(P_i)\,(RR - 1)}{1 + (P_i)\,(RR - 1)} \tag{8}$$

where n is the number of different risk factors and/or risk factor strata. This formula is provided for reference, but is not recommended for use in public health practice because it is extremely unlikely that common exposures will be mutually exclusive in a given context.

Although equations (6) and (7) are appropriate for estimating the contribution of multiple risk factors, they require information on joint exposures and associated relative risks. Such information is not commonly available, and in its absence, the most conservative approach is to use the largest AR associated with any single risk factor of interest. This approach will almost certainly underestimate the true AR, but if it is used consistently, it will produce results that can be legitimately compared.

Statistical Aspects

The variance of AR has received considerable attention since the mid-1970s.[2-8] The importance of confounding in estimating AR has been reviewed.[8] Methods for estimating ARs with multiple risks have been developed[9] and applied to the use of multiple logistic regression.[10-12]

PREVENTED FRACTION

Definition and Derivation

If exposure to preventive measure provides protection against acquiring a defined health problem (i.e., the associated RR is < 1), it is important to determine what proportion of the incidence of this health problem in a population is prevented by exposure to that preventive factor. Such protective factors may be intrinsic to an individual (e.g., the protection that the sickle cell trait is thought to provide against malaria) or extrinsic to an individual (e.g., vaccination). See "Comparing the Attributable Risk with the Prevented Fraction" below.

The *prevented fraction* (PF) is derived through the same logic used in deriving attributable risk (AR). That is, a simple definition of incidence is used, and issues of multiple exposures, study design, and confounding are ignored. In this context, the PF can be defined as the proportional difference between the incidence of a health problem in a population that does not have the protective factor (I_0) and the incidence of that health problem in a total population (including persons who do and do not have the protective factor) that does have the protective factor (I_T):

$$PF = \frac{I_o - I_T}{I_o} \qquad (9)$$

Substituting for I_T from the derivation of AF, the formula for PF becomes

$$PF = P_1 (1 - RR) \qquad (10)$$

Equation (10) expresses the PF in terms of the proportion of the population exposed to the protective factor (e.g., intervention strategy). The equation can also be expressed in terms of the proportion of persons who have the health problem and have also been exposed to the intervention:

$$PF = \frac{P_p (1 - RR)}{RR + P_p (1 - RR)} \qquad (11)$$

The proportion of disease that is prevented among persons who have been exposed to the preventive measure (PF_e) is the same formula that is commonly used to compute vaccine efficacy, i.e.,

$$PF_e = 1 - RR \qquad (12)$$

The prevented fraction of a health problem is the proportion of the incidence of a health problem in a population that has been prevented as a result of a *preventive factor* (intervention).

Statistical Aspects

Far less effort has been devoted to determining the variance of the PF than of the AR. Greenland derived a variance for PF in terms of PF_e.[7] Others have derived a maximum likelihood estimate for the PF for cross-sectional studies, and the result can be duplicated using the delta method.[13] There is no published method for determining confidence limits for PF.

IMPACT FRACTION

The concepts of AR and PF can be described with one formula:

$$IF = \frac{\sum_{i=0}^{n} (P_i - P'_i) RR_i}{\sum_{i=0}^{n} P_i RR_i} \tag{13}$$

in which P_i is the prevalence of the risk factor at the beginning of a given time period and P_i is the prevalence at the end of that time period.[14] When dealing with a causative exposure, and when P_i is considered to be the initial prevalence of the exposure, the formula reduces to the AR when $P'_i = 0$. Similarly, the meaning of exposure can be reversed, and if a preventive exposure is assessed in the same way, the formula will reduce to that for PF. This approach permits intermediate results to be evaluated, i.e., where $P'_i > 0$, and thus allows the impact of partial changes in the level of a risk factor or preventive measure to be evaluated.

A number of measures based on the IF are available for evaluating impact.[14] The *potential efficacy* of modifying risk factors can be expressed as the maximum number of potentially preventable cases divided by the number of persons exposed to an intervention, expressed mathematically as $AR/(1-p_0)$ (where p_0 is the proportion of the population not exposed to the risk factor of interest). The *potential effectiveness* is the expected number of preventable cases (based on the change that could be observed in the target population) divided by the number of persons exposed to the intervention; this relationship can be expressed as $IF/(1-p_0)$.

The *adequacy* of the intervention is described as the ratio of the expected number of potentially preventable cases to the number of cases that would occur in the absence of an intervention, and is equivalent to the IF itself. Finally, a more complex measure of *efficiency* is the ratio of the total number of preventable cases to the total number of persons expected to move to a category of lower risk.

Thus the impact fraction applies both to causation and prevention and can be used in comparing attribution in both situations. For purposes of presentation (and because the AR and PF are more familiar), it is of interest to compare the AR and PF directly in order to define the applicability of such measures to public health programs.

COMPARING THE ATTRIBUTABLE RISK WITH THE PREVENTED FRACTION

The AR and the PF are similar but not equivalent measures. The AR indicates the number or proportion of an outcome that would have been averted in the absence of an exposure that increases the likelihood of the outcome; or, conversely, the AR indicates the number or proportion of an outcome attributable to the exposure. The PF indicates the proportion of an outcome averted by the presence of an exposure that decreases the likelihood of the outcome; conversely, the PF indicates the number or proportion of an outcome prevented by the "exposure" (to a preventive measure).

In principle, the AR can be calculated for a preventive factor by inverting the meaning of exposure. Thus, those who are not exposed to the preventive factor are called the "exposed" group.[14] For example, in the context of a vaccination program, an exposed person is one who did not receive vaccine. With this inversion, the attributable risk among exposed persons ($AR_e = (RR - 1)/RR$) and the prevented fraction among exposed persons ($PE_e = 1 - RR$) are arithmetically equal, since the RRs used in calculating them are reciprocals.

SOME PRACTICAL CONSIDERATIONS

All measures of attribution can be easily misinterpreted. For example, it is legitimate to say that 80% to 90% of all lung cancer is attributable to smoking. However, this statement does not mean to imply that 80% to 90% of all cases of lung cancer would not occur if all smokers stopped smoking. Moreover, disease would not disappear immediately with the removal of an exposure because of the cumulative effects of that exposure over the years. Few, if any, exposures are susceptible to instantaneous removal. More important, the prevalence of exposure most often describes the current status of a process that has continued over time.

The AR actually estimates the proportion of a particular outcome, e.g., lung cancer, that would not have occurred if the population had never been exposed to a given risk factor, e.g., cigarette smoking. Despite the limitations of AR in calculating the effects of current risk factor control, the heuristic value of the measure—comparison of alternative public health scenarios, for example—may be substantial. If the AR (and by extension, the PF and IF) is to be used to advantage, several aspects to its calculation warrant examination.

Risk Factors and Preventive Measures

Attribution is only appropriate when the risk factor (or preventive measure) of interest can be assigned causality and when the magnitude of association (relative risk) has been assessed with proper regard for potential confounding factors (i.e., factors that distort the relationship between exposure and disease). Intermediate factors in a causal chain, or factors that alter the relationship of causal exposures to health problems (e.g., effect modifiers such as age) would not be appropriate candidates for attribution. For pragmatic rather than theoretical reasons, it can also be argued that attribution to nonmodifiable factors such as age and sex is irrelevant.

Prevalence of Exposure to Risk Factors

The instantaneous prevalence of an exposure in a population is, at best, conjectural. Clearly, prevalence is always an approximation, since it is measured over time (often substantial) and involves a dynamic population subject to immigration, emigration, mortality, and new cases of the health problem. For many health problems, these factors may be at equilibrium. However, for others, such as coronary heart disease and types of cancer whose incidence is changing rapidly, the prevalence of risk factors that contribute to changing incidence is also likely to be changing rapidly. More important, the prevalence needed for our calculation is the one that existed when persons who currently have the disease were exposed. For example, most current cases of lung cancer are related to the prevalence of smoking at least 15 years ago. Because of the persistent downward trend in smoking in the United States, use of data on current prevalence will lead to underestimates of the proportion of lung cancer that should be attributed to smoking. In contrast, coronary heart disease probably bears a more immediate relationship to smoking, and current disease may be more appropriately linked to current smoking prevalence. Thus the choice of exposure prevalence is not fixed but varies in accord with the relationship between exposure and health problem.

Relative Risks

The estimate of relative risks should be based on the same definition of exposure that is used to estimate prevalence. Definitions may vary for different data sets. For example, the prevalence of obesity in the U. S. population is often assessed from the second National Health and Nutrition Examination Survey (NHANES2)—a common source for many national risk-factor-prevalence estimates. In NHANES2, obesity is measured in terms of the Body Mass Index (the ratio of weight, in kilograms, to the height squared, in meters). In contrast, several studies, including that involving the well-known Framingham cohort, use the 1959 Metropolitan Relative Weight Tables and calculate the ratio of actual to "ideal" weight to obtain a measure of obesity. AR calculations using both sources would require equilibration of these measures.

In assessing relative risk, it is also important that variables have a constant meaning. Again, smoking provides a good example. The term *current smoker* is readily understood, but within populations there will be considerable individual variation with regard to quantity, type of inhalation, and frequency and duration of tobacco use. Populations, however, vary in their proportions of heavy smokers, inhalers, and occasional smokers, and this variation is probably related to the local smoking custom. Differences in the mix of exposures produce different estimates of relative risk.

Because the measure of relative risk describes the relationship of rates of a health problem in groups exposed and not exposed to the risk factor in question, different relative risks may also result from various rates in groups not exposed to the risk factor. In the case of cigarette smoking and lung cancer, the background rate (or referent used to calculate the relative risk) will be determined by the level of known and unknown carcinogens in the environment. A calculated relative risk is, strictly speaking, population-specific, although the similarity of certain relative risks across populations may indicate that the background rates for some diseases are relatively stable. Nonetheless, calculation of AR requires that both the prevalence and the relative risk be appropriate to the population of interest.

PUBLIC HEALTH IMPLICATIONS

When the preventive factor is extrinsic—when it is, for example, a public health intervention, both the strength of the intervention and, in particular, its prevalence, are to some extent under the control of a program. The PF (or the IF) provides a direct measure of the portion of disease prevention for which the public health program can take credit. Since, as noted, this portion of prevention will tend to be small for many chronic disease interventions, there is a certain honesty in this approach.

When evaluating prevention effectiveness, then, use of the PF provides a direct post hoc measure of benefits. Such benefits can then be expressed in terms of dollars or other measures, e.g., quality-adjusted life years. Costs of a public health program can be assessed and compared with the estimate of benefits that have accrued. If the IF is used, effects of increases in a preventive measure can be assessed, or potential benefit can be evaluated. Either approach provides more meaningful information than that associated with the simple question dealt with through the unadorned AR (i.e., What if there had been no exposure to this risk?).

REFERENCES

1. Levin ML. The occurrence of lung cancer in man. *Acta Union Intern Cancer* 1953;9:531–41.
2. Walter SD. The distribution of Levin's measure of attributable risk. *Biometrika* 1975;62:371–74.
3. Walter SD. The estimation and interpretation of attributable risk in health research. *Biometrics* 1976;32:829–49.
4. Walter SD. Calculation of attributable risk from epidemiological data. *Int J Epidemiol* 1978;7:175–82.
5. Whittemore AS. Statistical methods for estimating attributable risk from retrospective data. *Stat Med* 1982;1:229–43.
6. Leung HM, Kupper LL. Comparisons of confidence intervals for attributable risk. *Biometrics* 1981;37:293–302
7. Greenland S. Variance estimators for attributable fraction estimates consistent in both large strata and sparse data. *Stat Med* 1987;6:701–8.
8. Benichou J. Methods of adjustment for estimating the attributable risk in case-control studies: a review. *Stat Med* 1991;10:1753–73.
9. Bruzzi P, Green SB, Byar DP et al. Estimating the population attributable risk for multiple risk factors using case-control data. *Am J Epidemiol* 1985;122:904–14.
10. Coughlin SS, Nass CC, Pickle LW et al. Regression methods for estimating attributable risk in population-based case-control studies: a comparison of additive and multiplicative models. *Am J Epidemiol* 1991;133:305–13.

11. Drescher K, Schill W. Attributable risk estimation from case-control data via logistic regression. *Biometrics* 1991;47:1247–56.
12. Kooperberg C, Petitti DB. Using logistic regression to estimate the adjusted attributable risk of low birth weight in an unmatched case-control study. *Epidemiology* 1991;2:363–66.
13. Gargiullo PM, Rothenberg RB. Confidence intervals, hypothesis tests, and sample sizes for the prevented fraction in cross-sectional studies. *Stat Med* 1995;14:51–72.
14. Morgenstern H, Bursic ES. A method for using epidemiologic data to estimate the potential impact of an intervention on the health status of a target population. *J Community Health* 1982;7:292-309.

BIBLIOGRAPHY

Greenland S, Robins JM. Conceptual problems in the definition and interpretation of attributable fractions. *Am J Epidemiol* 1988;128:1185–97.
Kleinbaum DG, Kupper LL, Morgenstern H. *Epidemiologic research: principles and quantitative methods*. Belmont, CA: Lifetime Learning Publications, 1982.
Miettinen OS. Proportion of disease caused or prevented by a given exposure, trait or intervention. *Am J Epidemiol* 1974;99:325–32.
Park CB. Attributable risk for recurrent events. *Am J Epidemiol* 1981;113:491–93.

Appendix K
Meta-Analysis

REBECCA J. KLEMM
DONNA F. STROUP
G. DAVID WILLIAMSON

The breadth of research literature has made it practically impossible to keep abreast of all of the findings that are relevant to any given scientific discipline. Consequently, researchers rely heavily on published reviews of related literature to obtain the most up-to-date information relevant to their research interests. However, the rapid growth in available information has made the review process itself more demanding.

In sociological and biomedical research the reviewer will frequently discover conflicting research findings. The inclusion of more studies in the review does not usually resolve the problem, but rather adds additional discordant findings. While some of the disagreements in research findings across studies can be attributed to sampling error and differences in the definition and measurement of variables, the methodology used to synthesize the literature review may also contribute to the variations in study findings. Thus there is need for a more valid and reliable procedure for integrating possibly conflicting research findings than the traditional qualitative review. Such a procedure is provided by a set of quantitative techniques known as meta-analysis.

Public health is concerned with the prevention of unnecessary disease, injury, and disability and the promotion of a healthy community. Policy decisions in public health rely on results from studies from multiple disciplines, including clinical medicine, epidemiologic studies, laboratory research, statistical science, and behavioral theory. Thus the proliferation of published results in a given area is a particular problem in public health. In addition, in public health we have the ethical dilemma of taking appropriate action once a health problem is detected; such interventions cannot always wait for long-term, expensive clinical trials.

Meta-analysis is an objective, quantitative procedure for analyzing and synthesizing data or results from several independent studies. The studies must be "combinable" in some respect. In particular, they should have a commonality of at least one parameter of interest, for example, effect size, relative risk, or odds ratio. They must involve common study populations, homogeneity of outcomes, and sufficient reported information to be combined.

According to the National Library of Medicine, meta-analysis is a "quantitative method of combining the results of independent studies (usually drawn from the published literature) and synthesizing summaries and conclusions which may be used to evaluate therapeutic effectiveness, plan new studies, etc., with application chiefly in the areas of research and medicine" (National Library of Medicine, 1989).

In other words, meta-analysis serves to find, appraise, and combine data from a range of research to answer questions in ways individual studies cannot (Henry and Wilson, 1992). It can help to integrate research findings that seem to be inconsistent (Mottola, 1992).

The term *meta-analysis* was introduced in 1976 by Glass, who viewed it as the "analysis of analyses": and "aimed at the generalization and practical simplicity" (Glass et al., 1981). Glass categorized three types of research:

1. Primary analysis of the original analysis of data in study
2. Secondary analysis, which reanalyzes original data in order to answer the original question with more accurate statistical methods or to answer a new question
3. Meta-analysis, which integrates findings from numerous studies through quantitative means, using many methods of measurement and statistical analysis (Glass et al., 1981)

The work of Glass illustrated the "importance of systematically evaluating and synthesizing the results of independent tests of the same hypothesis" (Wolf, 1986) and widespread interest in meta-analysis resulted from his study. The procedure uses the "results of prior studies as its units of observation" (Abramson, 1990) and has gained recognition and acceptance in the past decade. Although some scientists have expressed skepticism about this technique, its consistency as a statistical measure is outweighing its potential drawbacks.

We present an overwiew of meta-analysis in epidemiologic research. Attention will be restricted to statistical approaches to the estimation of weighted averages of parameters of interest, such as treatment effects, relative risks, or odds ratios, across several independent studies. Qualitative aspects of meta-analysis, for example, procedures for collecting, coding, and organizing data for meta-analysis, are only mentioned for purposes of completeness. No attempt is made to treat thest topics in detail, because they are adequately covered elsewhere in the meta-analysis literature.

This appendix is structured as follows:

• In the first part we discuss some of the merits and criticisms of meta-analysis relative to the traditional narrative literature review. Our discussion includes some recommendations on how some of these criticisms can be addressed.
• The second part is a discussion of meta-analysis as a scientific process.

The reader is taken through a step-by-step description of the meta-analytic process, and these steps are shown to conform to the standard scientific method.

- In the third part we illustrate the use of meta-analysis in a variety of applications within the arena of public health.
- In the forth part, we present the general statistical methodology for meta-analysis. We adopt a general linear model approach to the estimation of overall treatment effects, relative risk, or odds ratios using estimates from several independent studies. In particular, we will discuss the fitting of parametric models to study-level estimates. Both fixed-effects and random-effects models will be presented.

MERITS AND CRITICISMS REGARDING META-ANALYSIS

Merits of Meta-Analysis

Until recently, the traditional narrative review was the preferred method for summarizing and synthesizing a group of studies. However, there are several drawbacks associated with this approach, including:

1. Subjective judgments, preferences, and biases of the reviewer, regarding the selection and weighting of studies, and the interpretation of the results of the analysis.
2. Failure to examine characteristics of the studies as potential explanations for disparate or consistent results across studies; and moderating variables in the relationship under examination.
3. Publication bias.
4. Bias of the reviewer to the outcome (i.e., desire of the reviewer to find significant or nonsignificant results).

When properly done, meta-analysis addresses some of the problems outlined above. What distinguishes a meta-analysis from a traditional narrative review is its quantitative nature and prescribed steps in methodology. Compared to a literature review, a meta-analysis "usually addresses sharper questions, usually with quantitative answers" (Louis et al., 1985, p. 2).

Each study provides estimates of effect and some measure of the accuracy of the estimates. Inferences are then based on rigorous statistical analysis of the study-level estimates. The quantitative nature of meta-analysis affords it a large range of utility. The merits of meta-analysis can be summarized as follows:

1. The combination of data from several sources has the potential for increasing the generalizability of the results and the statistical power for tests of hypotheses.
2. It is possible to test hypotheses about variables that differ among studies (subgroups) that generally would be difficult to test within a study. Exam-

ples of such variables are age, sex, level of education, degree of urbanization, and confounding risk factors.

3. Meta-analysis gives insight into the nature of relationships among variables and provides a mechanism for detecting and exploring apparent contradictions in results from single studies.
4. Meta-analysis enables us to detect heterogeneity of parameters of interest (treatment effects, relative risks, or odds ratios) and provide suggestions for searching for the cause of heterogeneity.

Criticisms of Meta-Analysis

There have been many criticisms of meta-analysis since it was introduced. However, a considerable number of these criticisms are induced by problems inherent in any literature review, rather than specifically with meta-analysis. Shortcomings of meta-analysis are often shortcomings of the primary studies. For instance, if problems with data quality, sampling bias, reporting, etc., exist in the primary studies, they cannot be resolved by meta-analysis.

Although the papers underlying a meta-analysis are based on experiments, observational studies, sample surveys, or other forms of investigation, the meta-analysis of these studies is an observational study. The meta-analyst differs from the investigator of a prospective primary study, in that he or she has control only over which studies to include, not what "treatments" were applied nor how "subjects" were selected and assigned (Louis et al., 1985).

The following is a list of the most commonly accepted criticisms of meta-analysis, as outlined by Glass et al. (1981):

1. Logical conclusions cannot be drawn by comparing and aggregating studies that include different measuring techniques, definitions of variables (e.g., treatments, outcomes), or subjects, because they are too dissimilar.
2. Results of meta-analysis may be uninterpretable because results from poorly designed studies are included along with results from well-designed studies.
3. Published research is biased in favor of significant findings, because nonsignificant findings are rarely published; this leads to biased meta-analysis results.
4. Multiple results from the same study are often used, which may bias or invalidate the meta-analysis and make the results appear more reliable than they really are, because these results are not independent.

Several measures can be taken to address these criticisms and, at the same time, maximize the benefits of meta-analysis. The first criticism can be circumvented empirically by coding the characteristics for each study and then applying statistical tests for differences among studies (heterogeneity).

The second criticism can be dealt with empirically by coding the quality of each study and statistically testing for differences in the results between poorly designed and well-designed studies (Thacker, 1988). The meta-analyst should be aware of the fact that even though there may be no significant differences in effect size between poorly designed and well-designed studies in a meta-analysis, there may be significant differences in the variance of effect sizes.

The third criticism can be addressed by expanding literature reviews to include research findings in books, dissertations, unpublished papers, or technical reports presented at professional meetings, etc., and comparing these results to those of published reports. Some of the literature argues against this approach, however, based on study quality.

Several approaches can be used to deal with the fourth criticism. For instance, separate analyses may be conducted for each different outcome tested. Alternatively, the meta-analyst may limit the number of results to be utilized from the studies to a fixed number and/or make adjustments for multi-collinearity.

META-ANALYSIS AS A SCIENTIFIC DISCIPLINE

In recent years, there has been considerable interest in the statistical methodology for meta-analysis, particularly in the areas of sociological and clinical research. The term *meta-analysis* was coined by Glass (1976), but research on the combination of data or results from several independent studies dates from as early as the 1930s.

Several authors, for instance, Cochran (1937), Yates and Cochran (1938), Cochran (1954), and Rao, Kaplan, and Cochran (1981) have described procedures for combining estimates from several different experiments to form an overall estimate. Hedges and Olkin (1985), and references cited therein, provide a detailed and comprehensive discussion of the statistical aspects of meta-analysis, and the applications of meta-analysis to various areas of research. Huque (1993) extended the earlier theoretical results of Cochran (1954) and others to the case when study-level covariates are incorporated in the analysis. Recent applications of meta-analysis have been illustrated by such authors as Antman et al. (1992) and DerSimonian et al. (1986) in randomized clincial trials; Fleiss (1991) in epidemiology and Bruvold (1993) and Thijs et al. (1993) in public health research.

Meta-analysis encompasses any systematic method that uses statistical methods for combining data from independent studies to obtain a summary measure of the effect of a particular variable (procedure) on a defined outcome (result) (Thacker, 1988). First used in psychology, it was adapted to the medical literature for randomized clinical trials and has been used more recently for nonrandomized epidemiologic studies. Among approaches to meta-analysis, generally six steps are used:

1. Defining the problem and criteria for admission of studies
2. Locating research studies
3. Classifying and coding study characteristics
4. Quantitatively measuring study characteristics on a common scale

5. Aggregating study findings and relating finding to study characteristics
6. Reporting the results (Cook et al., 1992)

Each of these steps presents particular issues in meta-analysis.

We discussed some of the commonly accepted criticisms of meta-analysis and how they might be addressed. We now suggest some guidelines for conducting meta-analysis in such a way as to take full advantage of the merits of meta-analysis while, at the same time, minimizing its shortcomings. Many conceptual and quantitative issues arise in the meta-analysis process and its is important that the analyst have a thorough understanding of the problem being investigated as well as of related issues. We follow the six steps identified above.

Step 1: Defining the Problem and Criteria for Admission of Studies

This is perhaps the most important part of doing a meta-analysis. It involves such conceptual issues as the formulation of the specific problem to be investigated, and the explicit definition of the treatment construct, the outcome and potentially confounding variables, and the criteria for inclusion or exclusion of studies.

For meta-analysis in general, the outcome of interest may take several different forms (Thompson, 1993). For example, studies of coffee consumption on the risk of coronary heart disease measure such heterogeneous outcomes as sudden cardiac death, myocardial infarction, coronary insufficiency, and angina pectoris (Greenland, 1987). In studies of the effect of low-level lead exposure on development, outcomes may be measured as percentage of children below a specified IQ level (Thacker, 1988). This variability in the definition of outcomes within or among studies presents difficulties when the results are combined in a meta-analysis.

In the selection of studies for inclusion, the specificity of the study question becomes critical (Fleiss, 1993). For example, in a study of the effect of estrogen replacement therapy on breast cancer, the country where the study was performed was important in study selection, since treatment regimens differed (Steinberg et al., 1991). Similarly, because studies may adopt different reporting categories (e.g., ever-use of estrogen rather than duration of use), selection of studies may be dependent on consideration of exposure variables as well as outcome.

Inclusion of only published research may bias the results of the meta-analysis, as the likelihood of being published is often reduced for "insignificant" results. Thus the meta-analyst must define the scope of research to review: books, published research, unpublished working papers, government studies, etc.

Step 2: Locating Research Studies

Once the meta-analyst has clearly formulated the research problem and clearly defined the research literature of interest, the next step involves implementing an effective strategy for locating and evaluating relevant studies. The goal of the literature search is to obtain an unbiased sample of the relevant studies by minimizing selective reporting and publication biases.

Among published studies, the task of study retrieval is complicated. Due to the complexity of medical and public health problems, relevant studies may be spread through a diverse literature, including nonmedical journals or government publications. For example, searches using MEDLINE may fail to identify relevant studies because of year of publication, consideration of limited interest, or publication in a journal of low circulation. In addition, the choice of search terms affects the inclusion of an article; one evaluation using a trials registry as the "gold standard" found only 32% of the relevant articles using MEDLINE (Petitti, 1994). Therefore, multiple search methods must be used in locating relevant studies for a meta-analysis. The steps are as follows:

1. Conduct both manual and computerized searches of indexing data bases (e.g., MEDLINE, TOXLINE, Index Medicus, Social Science Citation Index, Current Index to Statistics) and abstracting services (e.g., International Pharmaceutical Abstracts, University Microfilms), to obtain research articles and sources of both published and unpublished data.
2. Examine references cited in the studies located in (1) to obtain more studies.
3. Contact persons and organizations who are likely to have undertaken or to know of relevant studies.
4. Obtain nonrefereed reports and unpublished data from academic, private, and government researchers.

Step 3: Classifying and Coding Study Characteristics

Having selected the acceptable studies for a given problem, the reviewer develops a mechanism for classifying and coding study characteristics which might potentially influence the study findings. These include type of experimental condition, length of treatment, sample design characteristics, research design characteristics and quality, source of study (for instance, published, dissertation, internal/technical report, etc.), date of study, types of subjects, number of subjects, number of subjects in the various experimental and control groups, their means and standard deviations. It is better to code too many rather than too few categories.

Human error and multiple citing of the same information (e.g., in the abstract, results, table, and discussion) may lead to problems in this relatively straightforward procedure. Multiple publications of a single study increase the complexity of coding study characteristics.

Step 4: Quantitative Measuring of Study Characteristics on a Common Scale

The first step in the statistical analysis is to specify a method of quantitatively measuring study characteristics on a common scale. Furthermore, the various statistical outcomes in the studies of interest are converted into a common, quantitative metric, the index of effect, that can then be compared, aggregated, and analyzed across studies in the sample. The most commonly used index of effect in the social or biomedical sciences is the standardized effect size, which is the difference between the means of the experimental group and the control group, divided by a suitably chosen standard error. Frequently, this standard error is chosen to be the standard error of the control group, or the pooled standard error of the two groups.

The standardized effect size is an index of both the direction and magnitude of effect of a treatment or procedure under study. The statistical analysis of the data then focuses on the distribution of effect sizes and their covariation with the various descriptive variables coded in each study. For studies concerned with correlational association, the index of choice is a correlation coefficient.

Blinding of the abstractor to aspects of publication and results is perhaps the only reliable way of eliminating the problem of bias in data abstraction. Information in the report may not be presented in a useful way (e.g., risk estimates with the confidence intervals or variance necessary for analysis). Agreement among experts, for example, in the assessment of study quality, may be affected by training or expertise (Oxman and Guyatt, 1993).

Issues to be resolved by the analyst at this stage include choosing an outcome measure, deciding on a unit and model for analysis, and choosing an appropriate statistical method for analyzing the results. Technical details on statistical analysis for meta-analysis are provided later.

Step 5: Aggregating Study Findings and Relating Findings to Study Characteristics

The final stage in the meta-analysis process involves drawing appropriate conclusions based on the statistical analysis. The following guidelines should be taken into consideration at this stage.

1. Nonsignificant meta-analytic results may reflect the true state of affairs, but they may also be due to such factors as confounding variables that suppress real differences on the variables of interest, gross error in the primary data, and low statistical power due to, for instance, missing data, small cell sizes, etc. It is therefore recommended that meta-analytic results be throughly examined to establish that nonsignificant results are not simply due to confounding, poor data quality, or low statistical power.
2. Conclusions from meta-analysis should be restricted specifically to the literature reviewed. The issue of publication bias (increased probability of publication of studies reporting statistically significant results) has a differential effect across study designs.
3. The meta-analyst sould qualify results from meta-analysis in relation to the limitations of the available studies, particularly with restricted or diminished data on certain variables of interest. For example, it would be misleading to conclude that the length of treatment has no effect on

outcomes if the majority of studies involve short-term interventions of 10 sessions or less.

Sources of bias (or internal validity) affect the results of meta-analysis (Felson, 1992). For example, in studies of the health knowledge and attitudes of school children and the effect of desegregation, treatment and control groups are generally self-selected so that one group begins with a higher initial level (Bryant and Wortman, 1984).

Finally, it must be remembered that results and conclusions from meta-analysis are always subject to the quality of the primary data.

4. Cumulative meta-analysis is a technique that permits the identification of the year (or event in a series of time-ordered events) when the combined results of multiple studies first achieve and a priori level of statistical significance (Antman et al., 1993). Cumulative meta-analysis can also reveal whether a trend appears to be in favor of one intervention or another, or whether little difference in treatment effect can be expected. It allows investigators to assess the impact of each new study on the pooled estimate of the treatment effect.

Cumulative meta-analysis consists of a "time-series" of meta-analyses, where the meta-analysis is "updated" each time a new study or additional data are available. Cumulative analysis has stopped some randomized clinical trials of major medical, behavioral, and economic importance.

Step 6: Report the Results

EXAMPLES OF META-ANALYSIS IN THE PUBLIC HEALTH ARENA

In "Findings for Public Health from Meta-Analyses" Louis et al. (1985) illustrate examples of numerous meta-analyses studies regarding patient education and behavior modification (i.e., effects of psycho-education intervention on hospital length of stay), prevention (i.e., effectiveness of acidulated phospho fluoride gels and solutions and fluoride varnishes for prevention of caries), and epidemiologic studies (i.e., lead as a carcinogen).

From among the plethora of examples available in the literature, we provide three that illustrate the breadth of meta-analysis:

1. Adolescent smoking prevention programs
2. Oral contraceptives and the risk of gallbladder disease
3. Treatments for myocardial infarction

We provide a summary of the work reported in each of the three identified articles.

Adolescent Smoking Prevention Programs

William Bruvold, PhD performed a meta-analysis of adolescent smoking prevention programs. His work is presented in the June 1993 issue of the *American Journal of Public Health*.

212   APPENDIX K

Nonquantitative reviews of the literature had not focused on the following three questions/issues:

1. The general success of the programs
2. Whether program orientation is related to success
3. Identification of variables, other than program orientation, that relate to levels of success

Dr. Bruvold evaluated 94 separate interventions in his meta-analysis. Studies were screened for methodological rigor and those with weaker methodology were segregated from those with more defensible methodology. Most of his results are based on the latter group of studies. The subset of studies selected for his work was published during the 1970s and 1980s and dealt with the prevention of smoking in a school setting. Only college level settings were excluded.

His search involved checking the index issues of relevant journals to find appropriate studies. He then used the references in these papers to locate other germane papers. He conducted ERIC and MEDLINE computer-based searches and reviewed U. S. Department of Health and Human Services bibliographies on smoking and health. His search uncovered 141 articles, of which 84 were included in the meta-analysis. The reasons for setting aside 57 studies included: 27 because they were theoretical or review papers; 21 because they did not report on the evaluation of an intervention; and 9 because of problems with the comparison group. The resulting 84 studies met the three general criteria:

1. School-based program
2. Involved an evaluation of a program designed to prevent adolescent smoking
3. Included a comparison group that did not receive the organized program

Outcome measures were classified as falling into one of four time periods:

1. Immediate posttest
2. First follow-up
3. Second follow-up
4. Third follow-up

Effect sizes for behavior, attitude, and knowledge measures were computed for all studies reporting the required means and standard deviations according to the formula proposed by Glass et al., (1981).

A coding scheme developed by Rundall and Bruvold (1988) was used to systematically assess evaluation methodology regarding the five most prominent methodological features identified by the nonquantitative reviews. A three-level code was employed: value of 1 designated "exemplary"; value of 2 for "defensible"; and value of 3 indicated "unacceptable." Each study was independently evaluated by the same two researchers who had earlier assessed program orientation along five methodological dimensions. All disagreements were reconciled before the computation of study effect size began. The 48 studies without any ratings of 3 were used to form the major cumulative findings of the quantitative summary.

The results of the meta-analysis suggest that school-based programs should consider adopting interventions with a social reinforcement, social norms, or development orientation.

Oral Contraceptives and the Risk of Gallbladder Disease

The August 1993 issue of the *American Journal of Public Health* contains a meta-analysis performed by Drs. Carel Thijs and Paul Knipschild investigating oral contraceptives and the risk of gallbladder disease.

In the past 20 years conflicting studies have been published concerning the relationship between oral contraceptives and the risk of gallbladder disease. Studies conducted during the early portion of the 20-year time frame reported an increased risk of disease associated with oral contraceptive usage; later studies did not identify this association. The authors reported that the meta-analysis was undertaken to answer four questions:

1. Were the older studies systematically biased by design flaws? (or are the newer studies less valid?)
2. Was there a tendency at the time of the earlier studies to publish only "positive" results?
3. How should the evidence in the studies be weighted?
4. Are there explanations for the inconsistencies?

Drs. Thijs and Knipschild used MEDLINE and EXCERPTA MEDICA to identify publications from 1983 to 1992. Publications prior to 1983 were identified using references from later period publications. The authors restricted their review to controlled epidemiologic studies of noncancerous gallbladder disease. Twenty-five studies were identified in 27 publications. Four of the publications were initial/follow-up studies. All 25 studies were subjected to the authors' query concerning design flaw.

All studies were rated for design flaws (or internal validity) as measured by consideration of:

- Confounding by pregnancy
- Confounding by contraindication
- Confounding by biased detection of gallbladder disease
- Biased registration of oral contraceptive use

Nine studies were subsequently identified as lacking design flaws which would bias results.

All studies were examined for bias in the reporting of results. Reporting bias of various types was found in many of the published studies. The reporting biases within the publications cited included:

- Citing only statistically significant relationships when many relationships have been examined

- Citing only statistically significant relationships when many secondary analyses are performed on data collected for other purposes
- Publishing only results of "positive," low power studies when many more had been undertaken to confirm an adverse drug reaction.

No large-scale studies were found to exhibit publication bias. Overall six studies had neither design flaws nor publication biases, and these were examined for explanation as to inconsistencies in findings.

Results of the six studies were pooled and a pooled odds ratio was calculated. The conclusion drawn from the meta-analysis was that given weak effect between oral contraceptives and gallbladder disease, the changing formulas for oral contraceptives and the large efforts already expended in regard to this research effort, that the safety of new oral contraceptives be evaluated by studying bile saturation and biliary function rather than by waiting for gallbladder disease to develop.

Treatments for Myocardial Infarction

In their 1992 *JAMA* article, "Meta-analyses and reviews of therapies," Antman et al. examine the relationship between accumulating data from randomized control trials of treatments for myocardial infarction and recommendations of clinical experts writing textbooks and review articles.

The research team searched MEDLINE from 1966 to 1992 using the search strings of "myocardial infarction," "clinical trials," "multicenter studies," "double-blind method," "meta-analysis," and "random"; references from relevant articles and books; and English-language medical texts, manuals, and review articles on treatment of myocardial infarction. Studies were selected for inclusion in the meta-analysis if they were randomized clinical trials (RCT) of therapies for reducing the risk of total mortality in myocardial infarction. Review articles and chapters in textbooks concerning clinical management of patients with myocardial infarction were also considered.

Two authors read the material and recorded results; discrepancies were resolved by conference.

The research team performed a cumulative meta-analysis and compared the results with the recommendations of the experts for different treatments for myocardial infarction. They also visually compared a traditional meta-analysis conducted at the conclusion of all 17 RCTs with the results that would have been obtained had the meta-analysis been performed on a cumulative basis over time from 1972 through 1988.

They concluded that finding and analyzing all therapeutic trials in a given field has become such an onerous task that clinical experts need access to better data bases and new statistical procedures to allow them to summarize evidence in a timely manner. An example was thrombolytic drugs that were not recommended by more than half of the experts, even for specific indications, until 13 years after they could have been shown to be effective from a meta-analysis perspective. Six years passed between the time the first meta-analysis result suggesting a reduction in mortality by thrombolytic therapy was published (Stampfer et al., 1982) until a majority of reviewers recommended it for either routine or specific use. After 1985, when an approximately 20% reduction in the risk of death was established at the $p < .001$ level (odds ratio of 0.7, 95% CI of 0.69–0.90), 14 reviews still did not mention the treatment or felt it was still experimental. Alternatively, beta-blockers were recommended by some of the reviewers up to 12 years before the relative risk reduction in mortality of 11% (odds ratio of 0.89; 95% CI of 0.80–0.99) reached the $p < .05$ level in 1986.

STATISTICAL METHODOLOGY

In this section, we present the basic statistical methodology for meta-analysis. Even though the methods are applicable to a fairly general setting, they are by no means exhaustive. In other words, they do not provide a comprehensive treatment of every meta-analysis problem. We begin our discussion by describing some vote-counting procedures, and then present some basic ideas of fixed-effects and random-effects analysis.

Vote-Counting Procedures

Conventional vote-counting procedures are similar to nonparametric methods in statistical analysis. They use the results of tests of significance reported in a series of studies to draw conclusions about the existence of a significant treatment effect. The results of independent studies under consideration are classified into three categories:

1. Statistically significant in one direction
2. Statistically significant in the opposite direction
3. No statistical difference

The category receiving the most votes is declared the "winner," that is, the best estimate of the parameter of interest.

An alternative procedure for performing vote counts in meta-analyses is described by Hedges and Olkin (1983). It involves:

1. Counting the number of positive and negative results, regardless of significance
2. Applying the sign test (Binomial distribution with $p = 0.5$; e.g., toss of a fair coin) to determine if one direction appears in the literature more often than would be expected by chance

Note that even though the vote-counting method is intuitively appealing and easy to implement, it is no longer recommended in meta-analysis because of the poor statistical properties associated with its use. These include a low statistical power and hence a high probability of a Type II error (that is, the error committed by failing to reject the null hypothesis of no treatment effect, when in fact it is false). This leads to faulty inferences about treatment effects. In particular, the vote-counting method can be strongly biased toward the conclusion that the treatment has no effect (see Hedges and Olkin, 1985). Moreover, the bias is not reduced as the number of studies increases.

Pooling Methods

Pooling methods are methods by which data from several independent studies of a single subject are combined in a single analysis. There are three basic methods for pooling data:

1. Pooling observations or observational units (for instance, patients in health studies)
2. Pooling statistics, for instance, standardized effect sizes, odds ratios, and relative risks. An example of this method is the Cochran-Mantel-Haenszel procedure for combining estimates from several 2×2 tables
3. Pooling p-values (statistical tests of significance) For this method, we assume that the statistical tests to be combined have a continuous test statistic, which in turn leads to a p-value that is uniformly distributed. There are many ways of pooling p-values. They include Tippet (Uniform), Fisher (Inverse Chi-square), Inverse Normal, and Logit

Statistical Analysis

To perform a meta-analysis requires only an outcome measure or estimate of a common parameter of interest, y_i, (such as an absolute treatment difference, an odds ratio, or a relative risk), and its estimated within-study variance σ_i^2. Incorporating both the study-level estimate and estimated variance in the analysis may considerably reduce the effects of heterogeneity. The general procedure can be summarized as follows:

a. For the i-th study, $i = 1, \ldots , K$, we compute an unbiased estimate, y_i, of the parameter of interest θ, say, and the variance σ_i^2 of y_i.
b. We assign weight ω_i to study i, and compute the overall estimate of θ. This is usually a weighted sum or average of the study-level estimates, that is,

$$\hat{\theta} = \sum_{i=1}^{K} \omega_i Y_i$$

where

$$\sum_{i=1}^{K} \omega_i = 1.$$

Note:
(i) $\hat{\theta}$ is an unbiased estimator for θ.
(ii) Appropriate weighting of studies, when estimates are averaged across studies, ensures that studies yielding more precise estimates (e.g., those based on large sample sizes) or higher quality studies contribute more to the combined result.

c. The optimal estimator of θ is obtained by minimizing the variance of θ subject to the requirement that

$$\sum_{i=1}^{K} \omega_i = 1.$$

This is usually achieved by choosing the weights to be inversely proportional to the variance of the study-level estimates. Frequently, we choose

$$\omega_i = 1/\sigma^2_i.$$

Since the combining of heterogeneous studies or material is a frequently accepted threat to the validity of meta-analysis, it is important that the analysis be based on reasonable assumptions about the underlying effects.

Statistical Issues

We now describe two different approaches to statistical analysis in meta-analysis. What distinguishes the two approaches is the difference in the assumptions about the underlying effects: *fixed effects* and *random effects*. The appropriate method for estimating the overall estimate and its standard error depends on our assumptions about the study-level estimates.

A fixed-effects approach is predicated on the assumption that the studies are homogeneous and sampled from a single population. The random-effects approach separates within-study variability from between-study variability within a hierarchical structure of the observed data. Hedges and Olkin (1985) describe the fixed-effects approach and DerSimonian and Laird (1986) and Morris and Normand (1992) discuss the random-effects approach.

CONCLUSION

This appendix has provided an overview of meta-analysis: any systematic method that uses statistical methods for combining data from independent studies in order to obtain a summary measure of the effect of a particular variable (procedure) on a defined outcome (result).

We identified the common six steps to performing a meta-analysis. We summarized examples of meta-analysis in the public health arena. We encourage researchers of public health to embark on meta-analyses within their own areas of expertise. The Centers for Disease Control and Prevention is developing software for conducting meta-analysis which will assistanalysts.

BIBLIOGRAPHY

Abramson JH. Meta-analysis: a review of pros and cons. *Public Health Review* 1990; 18:1–47.

Antman EM et al. A comparison of results of meta-analysis of randomized control trials and recommendations of clinical experts, treatment of myocardial infarction. *JAMA* 1992;268:240–248.

Bruvold WH. A meta-analysis of adolescent smoking prevention programs. *Am J. Public Health* 1993;83:872–880.

Bryant FB, Wortman PM. Methodological issues in the meta-analysis of quasi-experiments. *Issues in data synthesis.* Yeaton and Wortman (eds). San Francisco: Jossey-Bass, 1984.

Cochran WG. Problems arising in the analysis of a series of similar experiments. *Journal of the Royal Statistical Society* (Suppl.) 1937;4:102–118.

Cochran WG. The combination of estimates from different experiments. *Biometrics* 1954;3:101–129.

Cook TC et al. *Meta-analysis for explanation: a casebook.* New York: Russell Sage Foundation, 1992.

DerSimonian R, Laird N. Meta-analysis in clinical trials. *Controlled Clinical Trials* 1986;7:177–188.

Felson DT. Bias in meta–analytic research. *J. Clin Epidemiol* 1992;45:885–92.

Fleiss JL. The statistical basis of meta-analysis. *Stat Methods in Med Research* 1993;2:121–46.

Fleiss JL, Gross AJ. Meta-analysis in epidemiology, with special reference to studies of the association between exposure to environmental tobacco smoke and lung cancer: a critique. *J. Clin Epidemiol* 1991;44:127–135.

Glass GV. Primary, secondary, and meta-analysis of research. *Education Review* 1976;6:3–8.

Glass GV. *Meta-analysis in social research.* London: Sage Publications, 1981.

Greenland S. Quantitative methods in the review of epidemiologic literature. *Epidemiol Rev* 1987;9:1–30.

Hedges LV, Olkin I. Regression models in research synthesis. *American Statistician,* 1983;37:137–140.

Hedges LV, Olkin I. *Statistical methods for meta-analysis.* New York: Academic Press, 1985.

Henry DA, Wilson A. Meta-analysis: part 1: an assessment of its aims, validity and reliability. *Medical J Aust* 1992;156:31–8.

Huque MF. A meta-analysis method for utilizing study-level covariate information from clinical trials. Draft pending publication, 1993.

Louis TA, Fineberg HV, Mosteller F. Findings for public health from meta-analysis. *Ann Rev Public Health* 1985;6:1–20.

Morris C, Normand S. Hierarchical models for combining information and for meta-analyses (with discussion). *Bayesian statistics.* Bernardo J, Berger J, David A, Smith A (eds). London: Oxford University Press, 1992:321–344.

Mottola CA. Synthesis of research findings through meta-analysis. *Decubitus* 1992; 5:48–50.

National Library of Medicine. Medical subject headings–annotated alphabet list. DHHS National Institutes for Health 1989:1–40.

Oxman AD, Guyatt Gh. The science of reviewing research. *Doing more good than harm: the evaluation of health care interventions.* Warren KS, Mosteller F (eds). New York: New York Academy of Sciences, 1993.

Petitti D. *Decision analysis and cost-effectiveness analysis.* New York: Oxford University Press, 1994.

Rao PSRS, Kaplan J, Cochran WG. Estimators for the one-way random effects model with unequal error variances. *Journal of the American Statistical Association* 1981;76:89–97.

Rundall TG, Bruvold WH. A meta-analysis of school-based smoking and alcohol use prevention programs. *Health Education Quarterly* 1988;15:317–334.

Stampher MJ et al. Effects of intravenous streptokinase on acute myocardial infarction: pooled results from randomized trials. *N Engl J Med* 1982;307:1180–1182.

Steinberg KK, Thacker SB, Smith SJ, Stroup DF, Zack MM, Flanders WD, Berkelman RL. A meta-analysis of the effect of estrogen replacement therapy on the risk of breast cancer. *JAMA* 1991;265:1985–1990.

Thacker SB. Meta-analysis: a quantitative approach to research integration. *JAMA* 1988;259:1685–1689.

Thijs C, Knipschild P. Oral contraceptives and the risk of gallbladder disease: a meta-analysis. *Am J. Public Health* 1993;83:1113–1120.

Thompson SG. Controversies in meta-analysis: the case of the trials of serum cholesterol reduction. *Stat Methods in Med Research* 1993;2:173–92.

Wolf FM. *Meta-analysis quantitative methods for research synthesis.* London: Sage Publications, 1986.

Yates F and Cochran WG. The analysis of groups of experiments. *Journal of Agricultural Sciences* 1938;28:556:580.

Index